Thank you for your support, Bobbie

"NEVER GIVE UP"
Mich Laughlin

UNTAPPED 60

How Resilience and Perseverance Inspire a Profound Shift in Perspective

By Michael D.N Laughlin
Featuring Jarrett Robertson

MAKE IT A GREAT DAY!
JR

UNTAPPED 60:
How Resilience and Perseverance inspire a Profound Shift in Perspective
www.untapped60.com
Copyright © 2024 Michael D.N. Laughlin

ISBN:

All rights reserved. No portion of this book may be reproduced mechanically, electronically, or by any other means, including photocopying, without permission of the publisher or author except in the case of brief quotations embodied in critical articles and reviews. It is illegal to copy this book, post it to a website, or distribute it by any other means without permission from the publisher or author.

Limits of Liability and Disclaimer of Warranty
The author and publisher shall not be liable for your misuse of the enclosed material. This book is strictly for informational and educational purposes only.

AI Assistance Disclosure

The content of this book is the original work and true autobiographical story and intellectual property of the authors. Every idea and word was conceived and penned by the authors.

There were instances in which the author collaborated with AI for options as to how best to continue, better chapter headings, titles, subtitles, and such.

However, to enhance readability and coherence, Artificial Intelligence (AI) was employed mostly for the following purposes:

- Refinement of language for clarity, consistency and accuracy
- Organizational improvements, including the structuring of content and the addition of major side headings
- Harmonization of voice, style, and vocabulary across the manuscript
- Generation of chapter summaries to provide concise overviews at the end of each chapter

While the AI's involvement was mostly for editing, clarity, readability, and organization purposes, the fundamental underlying content, insights, and expressions remain entirely the creation of the author.

The purpose of integrating AI was to present the authors' ideas in the most polished and accessible manner possible.

Dedication

To all those who have weathered storms, faced demons,
and emerged stronger on the other side.
To the ones who have felt the weight of the world upon their
shoulders yet found the courage to keep moving forward.
To the silent warriors battling unseen battles,
may you know that you are not alone.
To the ones who have loved and lost, whose hearts
bear the scars of profound grief and unimaginable loss.
To the firefighters, the first responders, the unsung heroes
who rush towards danger while others flee.
To the ones who have dared to dream, to hope, to believe
in brighter tomorrows even when darkness looms large.

May this book be a beacon of light in the darkest of nights, a
reminder that even in the depths of despair, there is hope.
May it serve as a testament to the resilience of the human spirit,
the power of love, and the strength found in community.
May it inspire you to keep fighting, to keep believing, to keep
dreaming, for within you lies the power to overcome any
obstacle, to rise above any challenge, and to emerge victorious.

You are heard. You are understood. You are appreciated.

With endless gratitude and unwavering hope
Make It A Great Day!
Mike and Jarrett

Table of Contents

Acknowledgments ix
Foreword xi
About the Authors xiii
Prologue xix

Chapter 1: Choosing Life in the Shadow of Death 1
Chapter 2: Goodbye Too Soon 33

Photos 62

Chapter 3: Broken, Mended, Unstoppable 89
Chapter 4: Unexpected Crossroads of Fate 125
Chapter 5: Never Stop Climbing 133

Acknowledgments

To all the amazing doctors, nurses, and staff at Kingston General Hospital (KGH), Providence Care, and St. Mary's of the Lake.

You all are the real-life superheroes who saved my life when I needed it most. I can't thank you enough for your kindness, skill, and hard work. You didn't just fix my body; you helped me find my way back to a life full of amazing things, like being a firefighter, getting married, and starting a family.

Even though I was scared and hurting, you were there, taking care of me with so much love and care. Because of you, I'm here today, living my dreams and making the most of every moment. In my book, *Untapped 60,* I want everyone to know just how incredible you are and how much you mean to me. Thank you from the bottom of my heart for being my heroes.

Foreword

As a former NHL hockey player and two-time Stanley Cup champion, I've faced my share of challenges and triumphs. Growing up in Lethbridge, Alberta, Canada, nothing was ever handed to me. I wasn't the biggest guy on the ice, but I knew how to fight, to persevere, and to push beyond my limits. Reading *Untapped 60* took me back to those raw, gritty moments—times when resilience and determination were my only options.

Untapped 60 is a story that resonates deeply with anyone who's had to overcome adversity. It's about pushing through the toughest times and finding strength in the most unexpected places. The author's journey is a powerful reminder that no matter how many times life knocks you down, there's always a way to get back up, to keep fighting, and to ultimately triumph.

What struck me most about this book is its honesty and vulnerability. The author doesn't shy away from the pain and the struggles, but instead, he dives headfirst into them, sharing every raw detail. It's this authenticity that makes *Untapped 60* not just a story, but a lifeline for anyone who's ever felt lost, broken, or beaten by life. It's a testament to the indomitable human spirit and the unyielding will to survive and thrive.

As someone who's had to prove himself time and time again, I found a kindred spirit in these pages. The book challenges us to look beyond our circumstances, to dig deep, and to find the untapped potential within us all. It's a story that pushes us to confront our fears, to embrace our vulnerabilities, and to come out stronger on the other side.

Untapped 60 isn't just about overcoming obstacles; it's about transforming them into opportunities for growth and self-discovery. It's about finding light in the darkest moments and using that light to guide us forward. This book is a beacon for anyone who's ever doubted their own strength or questioned their path.

I am proud to endorse *Untapped 60*. It's a journey that will inspire you, challenge you, and ultimately change you. It's a reminder that no matter how tough things get, there's always a way to rise above and achieve greatness. So, lace up, get ready, and let this incredible story show you what's possible when you refuse to give up.

Kris Versteeg - Former NHL athlete, 2x Stanley Cup Champion, Co-Founder of Klevr App, and Entrepreneur

About The Authors

Michael D.N. Laughlin embodies the spirit of resilience in the face of unimaginable adversity. As Canada's only above-knee full-time firefighter, his journey is one marked by astounding feats of courage and determination, punctuated by three harrowing brushes with mortality.

At the tender age of 26, Michael confronted the fragility of life first-hand when he endured a catastrophic accident, leaving his left leg and arm grievously injured. Through sheer willpower and the marvels of modern medicine, he defied the odds and returned to his cherished role as a firefighter, adorned with permanent reminders of his ordeal—metal plates, pins, and graft scars mapping his journey of survival.

In the aftermath of his 30th birthday celebration, Michael's world was shattered when he returned home to find his girlfriend had taken her own life, plunging him into a sea of grief and PTSD. Each moment became a painful reminder of her absence, testing his resolve like never before. With unwavering determination and the support of loved ones, he forged ahead, embracing the transformative power of love to navigate the darkest of days.

But that wasn't the end. Life, relentless in its tests, struck once more. In a twist of cruel fate, a collision with a deer sent Michael hurtling into a realm of agonizing pain and irreversible change. The aftermath of this calamity saw him emerge as an above-knee amputee, his body broken and spirit tested beyond measure. Yet, in the depths of despair, his resolve remained unshaken. With unwavering determination, he declared, 'I will be a firefighter again,' exhibiting a resilience that defied comprehension.

As he grappled with the physical and emotional aftermath of his ordeal, Michael found solace in his unwavering belief that adversity was merely a stepping stone to greatness. Amidst the echoes of loss and grief, he found the strength to rise, confronting his demons with a courage that knew no bounds. Battling through the shadows of addiction, he emerged victorious, his unwavering spirit a beacon of hope for all who encountered his story.

Through the trials of his journey, Michael discovered love in the most unexpected of places—a beacon of light amidst the darkness. His union with Angela, a testament to the indomitable power of the human spirit, brought newfound joy and purpose into his life. Embracing the role of fatherhood with open arms, he found fulfillment in the embrace of his newfound family.

Driven by a profound desire to pay forward the blessings he has received, Michael has embarked on a mission to empower others facing adversity. From his Limb Loss Fitness Program to his captivating public speaking engagements, he serves as a beacon of hope for all who dare to dream in the face of adversity.

In the wake of unimaginable tragedy, Michael D.N. Laughlin stands tall as a testament to the resilience of the human spirit—an indomitable force capable of transcending the darkest of days and emerging stronger on the other side. His story serves as a powerful reminder that within every setback lies the seed of opportunity, waiting to blossom in the light of unwavering determination.

At first glance, you might see a polished speaker, a financial expert, and a successful author. But peel back the layers, and you'll find a story of relentless resilience, unwavering determination, and an indomitable spirit that has triumphed against all odds.

Jarrett Robertson's journey began with a dream that seemed destined to shatter. Accepted into Brown University on a Division 1 hockey scholarship, he soared with anticipation. However, by 2003, the harsh reality hit hard— he was forced to take a year off due to academic struggles, a devastating blow that shook the very foundation of his aspirations.

But where others might have faltered, Jarrett found the strength to rise. Returning to Brown in 2004, he seized his second chance with a ferocity born from adversity. Graduating in 2006 with a degree in Human Development marked not just an academic achievement but a testament to resilience—a monumental comeback from the brink of defeat.

Yet, his journey was far from over. For three years, he lived the grueling life of a semi-pro hockey player, battling debt and uncertainty. But with each setback, he refused to yield. Life, however, seldom adheres to a linear trajectory. At 29, stranded at a Pennsylvania gas station with no means to continue the journey, the specter of adversity loomed large. Yet, it is in the crucible of such moments that resilience finds its voice.

Transitioning into the fitness industry in 2010, he forged a new path as a male physique competitor, defying odds and clinching victories in a realm where discipline and dedication reign supreme. Sponsored by leading supplement companies, and featured in prestigious fitness publications, perhaps this was a turning point, but life had more challenges in store.

Simultaneously in 2010, Jarrett entered the financial services industry, facing the daunting task of building a practice from scratch despite a lack of financial expertise and a history of poor decisions. Yet, he embraced the challenge head-on, driven by a desire to help others secure their financial well-being.

Jarrett faced the abyss and emerged stronger each time. Navigating the tumultuous currents of personal struggles—confronting familial trauma and alcoholism to grappling with the shadow of mental and emotional damage—instilled within him an unwavering resolve to confront life's challenges head-on.

Yet, amid the chaos of life, and over 25 relocations, his narrative is one of relentless pursuit, anchored in the belief that adversity is not an impediment but a catalyst for growth.

In 2016, he ascended to executive leadership within one of Canada's premier financial institutions, leveraging his experiences to shape a narrative of empathy, perseverance, and authentic leadership. The accolades that followed—earning the prestigious CFP® designation, becoming an Executive Circle member of the Financial Psychology Institute, a Psychology of Financial Planning Specialist, and being ordained as an officiant—serve as milestones in a journey marked by tenacity and fortitude.

In 2021, on the cusp of his 40th birthday, Jarrett penned his inaugural book, *Make It A Great Day,* a testament to the transformative power of optimism in the face of adversity. But perhaps the pinnacle of his journey and subsequent collaborations came in 2024, with luminaries such as FBI Negotiator Chris Voss and esteemed colleague Michael Laughlin culminated in the publication of *Empathetic Leadership* and *Untapped 60,* amplifying the message of resilience and perseverance to a global audience. These collaborations encapsulate the essence of his journey—forging connections, overcoming obstacles, and finding strength in vulnerability.

Through every twist and turn, he has embraced life's challenges with a smile, determined to find solutions and appreciate the journey. His story is not just one of success but of resilience, perseverance, and the unwavering belief that no dream is too big to conquer. As a speaker, Jarrett brings not just expertise but a lived experience that inspires others to embrace their journey and make every day a great one.

Prologue
Embracing the Journey

"Life is a journey, and if you fall in love with the journey, you will be in love forever."
- **Peter Hagerty**

To the profound journey of self-discovery that awaits you with open arms and steadfast determination. As you embark on this odyssey, recognize the untapped reservoirs of potential that reside within the depths of your consciousness. Within the pages of *Untapped 60,* we unveil the truth that a significant portion—upwards of 60%—of your human potential lies dormant, waiting to be unleashed and harnessed for your greatest good.

With hearts aglow with possibility, embrace the challenges that await you on this path with unyielding courage and unwavering conviction. It is through facing these trials head-on that you'll uncover the hidden gems of resilience, creativity, and inner strength that lie dormant within you, waiting to be unearthed.

As you navigate the twists and turns of life's labyrinthine journey, may you never lose sight of the transformative power of the human spirit. It is this indomitable force that propels you forward, even in the darkest of nights, illuminating your path with a radiant glow of hope and possibility.

Harness the boundless potential of your mind to shape your destiny and manifest your deepest desires. Through the power of intention and focused effort, you can tap into the vast reservoirs of creativity, innovation, and resilience that lie dormant within you, propelling you toward your loftiest aspirations.

As you immerse yourself in the pages of *Untapped 60,* may you feel a stirring within your soul—a whisper of possibility beckoning you to step into your fullest expression of self. It is through embracing your untapped potential that you unlock the door to a life of profound fulfillment, purpose, and joy.

Embark on this journey, heart ablaze, with possibility and mind open to the infinite potential that awaits you. For within the recesses of your being lies the key to unlocking your true greatness—and you shall soar to heights beyond your wildest dreams.

Chapter 1

Choosing Life in the Shadow of Death

"Life is either a daring adventure or nothing at all."
~ **Helen Keller**, American author and educator who overcame the adversity of being blind and deaf.

1

A Wild Ride Begins

Life is a lot like a soccer game, isn't it? Imagine yourself on the field, the grass beneath your feet, the sun beating down on your back. The game is in full swing, and the ball is constantly in motion, careening unpredictably across the pitch. You never quite know where it's going to bounce next, but one thing's for certain—you've got to be ready to kick it back.

Now, picture my life as that soccer ball, bouncing haphazardly through a series of unexpected twists and turns.

There have been moments of triumph, where I've felt like the star striker scoring the winning goal in the championship game. And then there have been moments of defeat, where I've found myself sprawled on the turf, wondering how I managed to miss the easiest shot of my life.

But through it all, I've learned to embrace the uncertainty, to channel my inner goalkeeper and stand ready to defend my dreams against whatever curveballs life decides to throw my way. Because just like in soccer, the game of life is not about avoiding the challenges—it's about facing them head-on, with courage, resilience, and a healthy dose of humor.

So here's to the beautiful game of life, with all its unexpected twists and turns. Who knows where the next bounce will take us? But one thing's for sure—we'll be ready to kick it back, no matter what.

The First Bounce

Ah, the adventures of a three-year-old mind, where every mundane car ride could potentially morph into a thrilling escapade. Picture this: the backseat of my mom's station wagon, a realm of endless possibilities (or so I thought at the time). But let's rewind a bit, shall we?

It was a day like any other—or so it seemed. The sun was shining, the birds were chirping, and I was bubbling with the restless energy that only a toddler possesses. But deep down, beneath the innocent facade of a child strapped into a car seat, a rebellion was brewing. You see, my sister and her friends were engaged in what I perceived to be the most captivating activity known to mankind: playing Barbies. And there I was, confined to the constraints of vehicular captivity. The injustice!

Have you ever experienced that wrenching feeling of having to leave the playground when the fun is still in full swing? That's precisely the emotional turmoil I was grappling with. So, as the wheels of the station wagon turned onto a dusty dirt path, a mischievous spark ignited within me. In a move as impulsive as a squirrel darting across a busy street, I made my decision—I was going back to the Barbies.

With the audacity that only a three-year-old can muster, I flung open the car door and took a leap of faith. In hindsight, it wasn't the most tactically sound decision. Instead of gracefully landing on my feet like a seasoned gymnast, fate had a different plan. My legs, unfortunately, found themselves in the path of the moving vehicle, and my head made an abrupt acquaintance with the unyielding ground.

In those heart-stopping moments, with adrenaline coursing through my veins like a raging river, my mom's panic was palpable. It was akin to watching a suspenseful scene unfold in a blockbuster movie—only this time, I was the star, and the stakes were alarmingly real. But fear not, dear reader, for my mom was not one to succumb to despair. With the swiftness of a superhero swooping in to save the day, she scooped me up and whisked me away to the nearest hospital.

Now, let me paint you a vivid picture of the chaos that ensued upon our arrival. Picture a beehive buzzing with activity, with doctors and nurses darting to and fro like diligent worker bees. All eyes were on me, the pint-sized protagonist of this medical melodrama. And what did they find? Much to everyone's relief, yours truly emerged relatively unscathed. Sure, there was a superficial gash on my noggin, but nothing a Band-Aid couldn't fix. And as for my legs? They seemed to possess an elasticity rivaling that of the bounciest rubber balls known to humankind.

But wait, there's more! When the kindly doctor inquired about my impromptu flight from the vehicle, I uttered the immortal words: "I wanted to play Barbies." It was a statement as innocently absurd as claiming to have scaled Mount Everest because you wanted to catch a glimpse of the Yeti. Ah, the logic of a child—a delightful blend of whimsy and utter perplexity.

So there you have it, the inaugural chapter in the saga of my childhood escapades. A tale of rebellion, resilience, and the enduring pursuit of Barbie-related bliss. And as I would soon come to learn, this was just the beginning of a lifetime filled with equally improbable adventures.

Onward to the Next Adventure

Let's fast forward through the whirlwind of childhood—a blur of hockey pucks whizzing through the air, footballs spiraling in perfect arcs—a symphony of sports that defined the essence of my youth. Always the eager participant, I was the one charging ahead, hungry for the next exhilarating play. But amidst the roar of the crowd and the thrill of competition, there existed another side of me—a wild spirit yearning for the rush of tearing through muddy trails on four-wheelers and the icy embrace of snowy landscapes on snowmobiles.

Then came 2007—a pivotal year in the narrative of my life. A year when my insatiable thirst for adventure came with a hefty price tag. But for now, let's leave that chapter bookmarked and turn our attention back to the present.

This, my friends, is not merely a tale of bumps and scrapes. It's a testament to the audacity of leaping into the unknown, with both feet firmly planted and hearts pounding with excitement. It's about embracing the unpredictability of life, diving headfirst into the fray, unyielding in our pursuit of the game, no matter what obstacles lie in our path. For life, much like a thrilling rollercoaster ride, is filled with twists and turns, loops and drops—and believe me, we were just getting started

The Turn of Fate

Have you ever found yourself consumed by an anticipation so palpable that it seems to permeate every fiber of your being? It's a sensation akin to standing on the precipice of an adventure, the mere thought of the impending experience dominating your thoughts and sparking an exhilarating rush of excitement. This was precisely the state of mind in which I found myself on that fateful night, as the allure of snowmobiling eclipsed even the most cherished of pastimes.

The anticipation was electric, crackling in the air like static before a storm, as I eagerly anticipated the thrill of navigating the wintry terrain under the cloak of darkness. It was a passion that stirred within me with an intensity matched only by the fervor of a sports fanatic awaiting the opening whistle of a championship game. Yet, in the grand scheme of life's pleasures, it was akin to being presented with the age-old dilemma of choosing between two equally enticing desserts.

For me, the allure of snowmobiling transcended mere recreation—it represented a symphony of adrenaline and exhilaration, a chance to embrace the raw beauty of nature and surrender to the freedom of the open wilderness. It was a pursuit fueled by a primal longing for adventure, an insatiable thirst for the unknown that beckoned with promises of untold excitement and exploration.

In hindsight, it's remarkable how a seemingly mundane activity can become imbued with such significance, transforming into a beacon of anticipation that illuminates the darkest of nights. It's a testament to the power of passion and the inexorable pull of adventure that ignites the soul and propels us towards the unknown with unwavering enthusiasm.

The Storm Unleashed

As darkness enveloped the landscape, the frigid embrace of the night seemed to penetrate every fiber of my being, while the relentless snowfall added to the sense of isolation, cloaking the world in a thick veil of white. Undeterred by the harsh conditions, fueled by the reckless enthusiasm of youth, I ignited the engine of my snowmobile, its roar piercing the eerie silence of the winter night.

With my friend's distant taillight serving as the only beacon of guidance amidst the swirling chaos, I embarked on a daring pursuit across the frozen expanse of the lake. It was a thrilling game of cat and mouse, each twist and turn amplifying the adrenaline coursing through my veins. Losing sight of my companion was not an option—his red glow symbolizing safety and camaraderie in the vast expanse of the snowy wilderness.

Yet, with every twist of the throttle, the elusive light seemed to dance just beyond my grasp, taunting me like a mirage in the desert of snow. The pursuit became a test of skill and endurance, a battle against the elements and the limitations of perception.

In those fleeting moments, as the engine roared beneath me and the wind whipped against my face, I felt an exhilarating sense of freedom and exhilaration. It was a reminder of the raw power of nature and the boundless spirit of adventure that courses through the veins of youth.

But beneath the surface of excitement lurked a subtle undercurrent of danger—a reminder of the inherent risks that accompany such daring escapades in the unforgiving wilderness. It was a delicate balance between thrill and caution, a tightrope walk between exhilaration and peril that defined the essence of the snow-covered landscape.

In the end, as the night stretched on and the snow continued to fall, I couldn't help but marvel at the sheer beauty and unpredictability of the winter wilderness. It was a journey that tested my courage and resilience, leaving an indelible mark on my soul—a testament to the enduring allure of adventure and the timeless majesty of the great outdoors.

The Catastrophic Collision

In a heartbeat, catastrophe loomed on the horizon—a solitary island emerging from the tumultuous sea of the storm like a phantom in the darkness. Caught off guard, I braced myself for the inevitable collision, a split-second decision met with a wave of resigned acceptance. Releasing my grip on the handlebars, I whispered to myself, 'I'm dead.'

As I hurtled towards the looming obstacles, time seemed to slow to a crawl, each passing moment stretched to its breaking point. It was a surreal experience, akin to threading the needle through a maze of towering trees, the world spinning in a dizzying whirlwind of motion around me. And then, as abruptly as it had begun, the chaos subsided, leaving me miraculously alive yet painfully aware of the damage inflicted upon my mangled leg.

The aftermath was a surreal tableau of agony and disbelief—a grotesque testament to the unforgiving laws of physics and the capricious whims of chance. The searing pain radiating from my shattered limb served as a stark reminder of the fragility of life and the arbitrary nature of fate.

In that moment of reckoning, I found myself grappling with the profound fragility of existence, confronting the stark reality of mortality in the face of overwhelming odds. It was a humbling reminder of the delicate balance between life and death, a testament to the resilience of the human spirit in the face of adversity.

Alone Amidst the Blizzard's Wrath

Picture the sheer terror that grips your heart when you find yourself stranded amidst the unforgiving wrath of a blizzard, isolated in the vast expanse of wilderness. With your leg mangled—femur snapped, tibia and fibula protruding through torn flesh—blood staining the pristine snow a stark crimson, you're left at the mercy of the bitter cold, its icy tendrils gnawing at your very core with relentless ferocity.

Desperation claws at your insides as you reach for your phone, only to be met with the deafening silence of a dead battery—a lifeline cruelly snuffed out at the precise moment of direst need. Frustration simmers beneath the surface, a volatile force akin to a dormant volcano on the brink of eruption. Yet, amidst the swirling maelstrom of despair, a glimmer of hope emerges—a solitary cottage, its warm glow cutting through the icy darkness like a beacon of salvation.

As you fix your gaze upon this solitary haven, a surge of determination courses through your veins, igniting a flicker of optimism amidst the overwhelming chaos. With each labored step towards the distant refuge, you cling to the belief that within those four walls lies the promise of warmth, safety, and perhaps, a chance at survival.

In that fleeting moment, the boundaries between despair and hope blur into insignificance, as the primal instinct for self-preservation propels you forward, despite the insurmountable odds stacked against you. It is a testament to the resilience of the human spirit, forged in the crucible of adversity, and illuminated by the guiding light of hope in the darkest of nights.

The Perilous Journey to Safety

With each agonizing inch I crawled through the unforgiving terrain blanketed in treacherous snow, the searing pain in my shattered leg threatened to unravel my resolve like delicate strands of thread. It was as if every movement only served to amplify the relentless torment, each tug and pull on my fractured femur a stark reminder of the fragility of my physical being.

Twice, amidst the biting chill of the blizzard's icy embrace, I found myself sprawled on the ground, overcome by a profound sense of despair. In those fleeting moments, as the bitter wind howled around me, the thought of succumbing to the relentless grip of death crept insidiously into my consciousness. 'Just die,' I whispered to myself, the words a desperate plea born of sheer exhaustion and agony.

Yet, in the depths of my despair, something remarkable transpired. As I teetered on the precipice of surrender, a sudden surge of clarity pierced through the fog of hopelessness. It was the thought of my family and friends—the unwavering pillars of support amidst the tumultuous tempest of uncertainty—that ignited a flicker of resilience within me.

Their steadfast belief in my strength and unwavering perception of me as the resilient 'tough guy' became an indomitable force, propelling me forward against the tide of despair. How could I, in good conscience, allow myself to falter and disappoint those who had placed their faith in my fortitude?

In that defining moment, amidst the stark beauty and unforgiving brutality of nature's embrace, I found a newfound sense of purpose—an unyielding determination to persevere against the seemingly insurmountable odds. It was a testament to the transformative power of love, belief, and the unwavering support of those who anchor us in the stormiest seas of life

The Miraculous Rescue

Just when all hope seemed lost, the distant hum of a snowmobile engine shattered the oppressive silence—a lifeline thrown from the heavens in my darkest hour of need. My friend, gripped by a mixture of fear and disbelief, stumbled upon the scene, his eyes wide with shock at the sight of my broken form. But even amidst the throes of agony, I remained steadfast, issuing terse commands through gritted teeth, guiding him through the chaotic ordeal with the steely resolve of a seasoned commander on the battlefield.

"Help me get on the back of the Skidoo. I'm going to scream and yell the entire time for you to stop and act like every snowflake is a boulder that we're driving over. Listen to me, DO NOT STOP!"

The Ordeal Continues

The trials were far from over. As we wrestled with the logistical nightmare of transporting my injured body to safety, each obstacle seemed insurmountable—a Herculean task compounded by the excruciating pain coursing through my shattered limb. And as we raced against time towards the sanctuary of the hospital, every passing second felt like an eternity—a harrowing journey through the abyssal depths of uncertainty and despair.

In Retrospect

What transpired that fateful night transcended the realm of mere accident—it was a crucible of character, a trial by fire that tested the very fabric of my being. And through it all, one truth remained immutable: the indomitable spirit of resilience, burning bright amidst the darkest of nights, for surrender was never an option in the grand tapestry of life's unpredictable journey.

A Rush to the Hospital

Picture the world around you fading into a kaleidoscope of movement, each heartbeat pulsating in harmony with the urgent cadence of chaos. That's precisely how it felt as I found myself whisked away to the emergency room—a whirlwind of activity that seemed to mirror the relentless march of ants defending their besieged hill.

In that moment, the bustling energy of the medical team enveloped me like a protective cocoon, their movements synchronized with a precision that bordered on miraculous. Doctors and nurses darted around me with an unwavering sense of purpose, their every action imbued with a gravity that transcended the confines of time itself. It was as if the world had been thrust into fast-forward, every second ticking by in a frantic blur of urgency and determination.

Amidst the flurry of activity, I couldn't help but marvel at the sheer dedication and expertise on display—a symphony of skill and compassion orchestrated amidst the chaos of crisis. Each member of the medical team seemed to possess an innate understanding of their role in the grand tapestry of care, their collective efforts weaving together seamlessly to ensure my well-being.

As I lay amidst the whirlwind of motion, I found solace in the knowledge that I was in capable hands—surrounded by a team of professionals whose commitment to healing transcended the frenetic pace of the emergency room. It was a moment of profound realization, underscoring the profound impact of human connection and expertise in the face of adversity.

The Unforeseen Twist

There I lay, feeling exposed and vulnerable in the sterile hospital environment, draped in a flimsy gown that fluttered like a tattered flag in the breeze. Little did I anticipate the unexpected encounter awaiting me—the arrival of a nurse armed with the dreaded catheter, transforming what I thought would be a routine Band-Aid fix into an unwelcome surprise.

Caught off guard by the sudden intrusion, my reflexes kicked in, and I inadvertently sent the nurse stumbling backward, her surprise mirrored in my own eyes. Despite the unintentional commotion, she remained remarkably composed, her chuckle carrying a hint of understanding borne from countless similar encounters. With a reassuring nod, she excused herself from the room, promising to return momentarily.

A short while later, she reappeared, accompanied by a team of stewards prepared to tackle the seemingly innocuous procedure. It became evident that resistance was futile; the catheter was to be inserted, whether I welcomed it or not. As the sensation of discomfort washed over me, I couldn't help but liken it to enduring the most agonizing tickle—a fleeting discomfort masked by the gravity of the situation.

In that moment, I was reminded of the delicate balance between vulnerability and resilience, as well as the unwavering dedication of healthcare professionals tasked with navigating the complexities of patient care. It was a humbling experience, serving as a poignant reminder of the inherent vulnerability inherent in the human condition, and the remarkable fortitude required to navigate moments of discomfort and uncertainty.

Surgery and Revelation

Awakening from the hazy fog of anesthesia, I found myself confronted with a disconcerting sight—a formidable cast encasing my injured limbs, serving as a stark visual reminder of the gravity of my situation. The revelation of an additional cast on my arm sent a jolt of disbelief coursing through me, highlighting the profound capacity of the human mind to overlook the signs of impending danger in the relentless pursuit of our ambitions.

Much like a determined soccer player, singularly focused on netting a goal, oblivious to the loss of a vital component like their shoe, I too had become blind to the warning signals of my own physical distress. In a moment of disbelief, I turned to my mother, questioning the inexplicable presence of a cast on my arm, unaware of the extent of my injuries. The memory of my inquiry, 'What is wrong with my arm? How could it possibly be broken?' reverberated with a haunting clarity, as I recounted the events leading up to the accident.

In hindsight, this moment served as a poignant reminder of the inherent vulnerability of the human condition and the fallibility of our perceptions. It underscored the importance of mindfulness and self-awareness, urging me to heed the subtle whispers of my body amidst the cacophony of life's ambitions. It was a humbling revelation, shedding light on the delicate balance between determination and self-preservation, and prompting a profound reassessment of my priorities and perceptions.

The Arduous Journey of Recovery

Recovery, as I soon discovered, unfolded as a formidable odyssey riddled with trials—a veritable baptism of fire that demanded unyielding resilience and unwavering determination. Under the guidance of skilled therapists, I embarked on a journey fraught with challenges, the foremost of which involved reclaiming the most rudimentary of human movements—walking.

Each step I took resembled a Herculean ascent, akin to scaling the lofty peaks of a mountain range, albeit commencing from the modest foothills of my own backyard. The process was humbling in its entirety, reminiscent of the tentative ventures of a novice cyclist learning to balance on two wheels anew. Yet, with every cautious stride, I bore witness to the remarkable resilience ingrained within the human spirit—a testament to its unparalleled capacity for adaptation and growth.

Navigating this labyrinthine path of rehabilitation, I found myself grappling not only with the physical demands of recovery but also with the profound emotional and psychological toll it exacted. Each stumble served as a stark reminder of the fragility of the human condition, while every small victory echoed as a resounding testament to the tenacity and fortitude inherent within us all.

In retrospect, the journey of recovery transcended the mere reacquisition of motor skills—it emerged as a profound exploration of the resilience of the human spirit, an unwavering testament to our innate capacity for transformation and renewal. It was a voyage marked by setbacks and triumphs, ultimately culminating in a newfound appreciation for the remarkable resilience that resides within each of us.

The Power of Mind Over Matter

In the midst of grappling with physical discomfort and confronting psychological hurdles, I found myself stumbling upon a revelation so profound that it seemed to border on the miraculous. It was during this tumultuous period that I came to a profound realization: the incredible dominion of the mind over the body. Despite the admonitions urging me to abandon the telltale signs of weakness embodied in a limp, I unearthed an extraordinary truth—our brains possess an astonishing capacity to shape the very essence of our existence.

In that pivotal moment, I experienced a transformative shift in perception that defied conventional wisdom. Through a subtle yet profound alteration in mindset, I summoned the courage to banish the looming specter of limping from my gait. It was a testament to the immense power wielded by the mind over the constraints of physical reality.

This revelation illuminated the profound interconnectedness between our thoughts and our physical experiences, unveiling the latent potential residing within each of us. It underscored the pivotal role played by our mental fortitude in shaping the trajectory of our lives, even amidst the most challenging circumstances.

In essence, I learned that true strength lies not merely in the physical prowess we exhibit, but rather in the resilience of our minds and our unwavering determination to transcend perceived limitations. It was a journey that affirmed the boundless potential inherent within each of us, awaiting only the spark of realization to ignite its transformative flame.

Amygdala Hijacking

Amygdala hijacking is a fascinating concept that sheds light on the intricate interplay between our emotions and decision-making processes. Essentially, when we encounter a stimulus that triggers an emotional response, such as anger, fear, or frustration, the amygdala, a region of the brain responsible for processing emotions, can become "hijacked" or overwhelmed. This hijacking occurs because the amygdala perceives a threat, whether real or perceived, and initiates a rapid and intense emotional reaction.

As you've likely experienced, amygdala hijacking can manifest in various situations, from personal interactions to professional environments. Have you ever found yourself reacting impulsively to a comment or situation, only to later regret your response? That's a classic example of amygdala hijacking in action. In these moments, our emotions take the driver's seat, often leading to irrational or disproportionate reactions.

Understanding the psychological impacts of amygdala hijacking is crucial for navigating challenging situations effectively. When the amygdala is in control, it can override rational thinking and lead us to make decisions based on emotion rather than logic. This can result in impulsive behavior, conflict escalation, and poor judgment, ultimately hindering our ability to resolve conflicts or make sound choices.

Reflecting on your own experiences, you may recognize instances where amygdala hijacking played a significant role in your response to adversity. For example, when faced with the profound loss of a loved one or the challenges of addiction, the emotional intensity of these experiences likely triggered amygdala hijacking, influencing your actions and decisions.

In your journey, you've undoubtedly encountered moments where amygdala hijacking threatened to derail your progress.

For me, as an example, turning to painkillers as a coping mechanism in the face of emotional pain is a poignant example of how the amygdala's response to distress can lead to maladaptive behaviors. However, it's important to acknowledge that despite these challenges, you and I ultimately retained agency over our decisions.

The key takeaway from understanding amygdala hijacking is recognizing that while our emotions may exert a powerful influence, we still have the capacity to exercise control over our responses. This realization empowers us to develop strategies for managing emotional reactivity, such as mindfulness, self-awareness, and cognitive reframing.

In my journey of overcoming adversity, I've demonstrated resilience by actively engaging in behaviors that mitigate the impact of amygdala hijacking. Seeking help, acknowledging and owning my decisions, and cultivating a positive perspective are all examples of how I've reclaimed agency over my emotional responses. By acknowledging the role of amygdala hijacking in your experiences, you can continue to navigate life's challenges with greater awareness and resilience.

In conclusion, amygdala hijacking is a powerful phenomenon that underscores the complex relationship between emotions and decision-making. By understanding its psychological implications and recognizing our capacity for self-regulation, we can navigate adversity with greater resilience and agency. Your journey serves as a testament to the transformative power of acknowledging and overcoming amygdala hijacking, paving the way for personal growth and emotional well-being.

The Triumph of Resilience

Eight months had passed since the defining moment that forever altered the trajectory of my life. Standing at the threshold of the fire station, I couldn't help but marvel at the journey that had brought me to this point—a journey marked by trials, tribulations, and, ultimately, triumph over adversity. Like a phoenix rising from the ashes, I found myself poised to embrace life's challenges with a newfound sense of resilience and determination.

With each step forward, I felt the weight of my past struggles lift from my shoulders, replaced by a renewed vigor and a steely resolve to reclaim all that had once seemed lost. It was a moment of profound transformation, a testament to the indomitable spirit that resides within each of us, waiting to be unleashed in the face of adversity.

As I returned to the hockey rink and softball field, I did so with a sense of pride and purpose, each stride serving as a testament to the resilience of the human spirit. It was as though my leg, once broken and battered, had been bestowed with a reset button—a chance to start anew and rewrite the narrative of my life.

Yet, just as I began to settle into a semblance of normalcy, life, in its infinite caprice, saw fit to hurl yet another curveball in my direction. It was a stark reminder of the unpredictable nature of existence, a testament to the enduring quest for purpose amidst life's ever-unfolding twists and turns.

But through it all, I remained steadfast in my belief that every challenge is an opportunity in disguise—a chance to unearth hidden reserves of strength, resilience, and determination. And so, dear reader, as I embark on the next chapter of my journey, I do so with a sense of anticipation and curiosity, eager to see where life's unpredictable path may lead.

The Brain's Response to Trauma

Groundbreaking research within the realm of neuroscience affirms the profound symbiosis between our mental and physical states, elucidating the intricate mechanisms that govern the brain's response to trauma. Delving deep into the labyrinthine corridors of neural pathways, studies unveil the profound impact of traumatic events, not only on our physical well-being but also on the very fabric of our emotional landscape.

It's fascinating to uncover how the brain, in its remarkable adaptability, undergoes profound transformations in the wake of trauma. These changes extend beyond mere perception, as traumatic experiences have been shown to induce tangible alterations in neural pathways, reconfiguring the way we interpret and process pain. Moreover, the emotional responses triggered by such events are deeply intertwined with our perception of pain, creating a complex interplay between mind and body.

Indeed, our minds are adept at navigating the intricate dance between emotions and decision-making, often prioritizing self-preservation above all else. In times of distress, our brains instinctively resort to a primal instinct for survival, making decisions that are driven by emotions rather than logic. This phenomenon, known as the 'fight or flight' response, can lead us to adopt behaviors aimed at mitigating perceived threats, even if they may not always be rational or beneficial in the long run. Ever met someone afraid of flying? It's the safest form of travel in the world.

However, it's crucial to recognize that while our emotions may guide our initial reactions to trauma, they need not dictate our long-term trajectory. By acknowledging and processing our emotions in a healthy manner, we empower ourselves to transcend the constraints of instinctive responses and embrace proactive measures for healing and growth.

One effective strategy involves cultivating mindfulness—a practice that encourages us to observe our thoughts and emotions with detached awareness, without judgment or attachment. Through mindfulness techniques such as deep breathing, meditation, and self-reflection, we can gain greater insight into our emotional landscape and develop the resilience needed to navigate life's challenges with grace and equanimity.

Additionally, seeking support from trusted friends, family members, or mental health professionals can provide invaluable assistance in processing trauma and developing healthy coping mechanisms. By fostering a supportive network of individuals who understand and empathize with our experiences, we create a safe space for healing and growth.

Ultimately, while the impact of trauma on the mind and body may be profound, it's important to remember that we possess the inherent capacity to overcome adversity and emerge stronger on the other side. By embracing our emotions, cultivating mindfulness, and seeking support when needed, we can navigate the journey of healing with courage, resilience, and hope.

The Power of Perception

Embedded within the tumultuous storm of trauma, there exists a subtle yet undeniable glimmer of hope—a beacon of light that beckons from the recesses of our consciousness. It is within this realm of perception that the true transformative power of the mind unveils itself, offering a pathway towards healing and resilience amidst the darkest of times.

Research within the field of psychology and neuroscience has shed light on the remarkable influence of perception on our experience of pain and suffering. One seminal study conducted by researchers at Stanford University explored the phenomenon of placebo analgesia, wherein individuals experience a reduction in pain simply through the belief that they are receiving an effective treatment. This groundbreaking research underscores the profound connection between mind and body, demonstrating how our perceptions and beliefs can directly impact our physical sensations.

Consider, for example, the placebo effect in the context of pain management. When individuals are administered a placebo—a substance devoid of any pharmacological properties—but are led to believe that it is a potent pain reliever, they often report a significant reduction in their subjective experience of pain. This remarkable phenomenon highlights the power of perception to modulate our physiological responses, offering tangible evidence of the mind's ability to influence our perception of discomfort and distress.

Moreover, our perceptions extend beyond the realm of physical sensations to encompass our emotional experiences as well. Studies have shown that individuals who adopt a positive outlook and cultivate resilience in the face of adversity are better equipped to cope with stress and trauma. By reframing their perceptions of challenging situations and focusing on opportunities for growth and learning, these individuals are able to navigate life's obstacles with greater ease and resilience.

In essence, the power of perception lies in its ability to shape our reality and influence our responses to the world around us. By harnessing the innate potential within us to cultivate a positive mindset and resilient outlook, we can transcend the limitations imposed by physical pain and emotional anguish, paving the way for profound transformation and healing.

In our everyday lives, we can witness the impact of perception through simple yet profound examples. Consider the experience of receiving a compliment from a friend or loved one. In that moment, our perception of ourselves and our worth is elevated, leading to feelings of validation and self-confidence. Similarly, when faced with a challenging situation, such as a setback at work or a disagreement with a loved one, our perception of the event can either exacerbate our distress or provide a pathway towards resolution and growth.

Ultimately, the power of perception offers us a potent tool for navigating the complexities of life with grace and resilience. By cultivating a mindset of optimism, resilience, and self-awareness, we can harness the transformative potential of our minds to effect positive change in our lives and the lives of those around us.

Empowering the Human Spirit

Throughout the annals of human history, narratives of resilience and triumph have stood as enduring testaments to the unyielding strength of the human spirit. In the face of adversity and hardship, individuals from all walks of life have risen above their circumstances, defying the odds and forging paths towards a brighter tomorrow. These stories, woven into the fabric of our collective consciousness, serve as beacons of hope and inspiration, reminding us of the boundless potential that resides within each and every one of us.

Research within the realm of positive psychology offers valuable insights into the transformative power of optimism and resilience, shedding light on the ways in which these psychological constructs can shape our lived experiences and propel us towards self-actualization and personal fulfillment. One seminal study conducted by psychologist Martin Seligman explored the concept of learned helplessness and its counterpart, learned optimism. Through his research, Seligman demonstrated that individuals who cultivate a mindset of optimism are better equipped to overcome obstacles and bounce back from setbacks, ultimately leading more fulfilling and successful lives.

Consider, for instance, the story of Helen Keller, a remarkable individual who overcame profound challenges to become an influential author and activist. Despite being deaf and blind from a young age, Keller's unwavering determination and resilience enabled her to transcend her disabilities and make significant contributions to society. Her life serves as a poignant example of the power of optimism and resilience to surmount even the most formidable obstacles.

In our everyday lives, we can witness the transformative effects of positive psychology in action. Take, for example, the practice of gratitude—a cornerstone of positive psychology that involves acknowledging and appreciating the blessings in our lives. Research has shown that cultivating a gratitude mindset can lead to improved mental health, greater resilience, and enhanced overall well-being. By focusing on the positives in our lives, even amidst adversity, we can reframe our perceptions and foster a greater sense of happiness and fulfillment.

Moreover, positive psychology empowers individuals to harness their strengths and cultivate a sense of purpose and meaning in life. By identifying and leveraging their unique talents and abilities, individuals can tap into their full potential and pursue goals that align with their values and aspirations. This proactive approach to personal growth fosters a sense of agency and empowerment, enabling individuals to navigate life's challenges with confidence and resilience.

In essence, the principles of positive psychology offer us a roadmap for cultivating resilience, optimism, and fulfillment in our lives. By embracing these principles and adopting a mindset of growth and possibility, we can unlock the inherent potential within us and chart a course toward a brighter, more fulfilling future.

Cultivating Resilience

Resilience, much like a muscle, requires intentional effort and consistent practice to strengthen and sustain. It is not merely an innate trait but a skill that can be cultivated and nurtured over time. In the face of life's inevitable challenges and adversities, individuals who possess resilience demonstrate an extraordinary ability to bounce back and thrive. Research in the field of psychology underscores the importance of resilience in promoting mental well-being and enhancing overall quality of life.

One study conducted by psychologist Ann Masten explored the concept of resilience in children facing adverse circumstances such as poverty, trauma, and family dysfunction. Through her research, Masten identified several key factors that contribute to resilience, including supportive relationships, adaptive coping strategies, and a sense of purpose and meaning in life. These findings highlight the crucial role of resilience in fostering positive outcomes, even in the most challenging of circumstances.

In our daily lives, there are various strategies we can employ to cultivate resilience and bolster our mental fortitude. Mindfulness meditation, for example, has been shown to reduce stress, enhance emotional regulation, and promote overall well-being. By practicing mindfulness, we learn to cultivate present-moment awareness and cultivate a sense of inner peace and calm, even amidst life's storms.

Another effective approach is cognitive-behavioral therapy (CBT), a widely researched and empirically supported intervention for building resilience and promoting mental health. CBT helps individuals identify and challenge negative thought patterns and beliefs, replacing them with more adaptive and empowering alternatives. Through this process, individuals learn to develop resilience by reframing their perceptions and adopting a more positive and proactive mindset.

Furthermore, practices such as gratitude journaling can also contribute to resilience by fostering a sense of appreciation for the blessings in our lives. By regularly acknowledging and reflecting on the things we are grateful for, we cultivate a mindset of abundance and resilience, even in the face of adversity.

Real-life stories of human resilience serve as powerful reminders of the transformative power of resilience in overcoming life's challenges. Take, for instance, the story of Malala Yousafzai, a Pakistani activist who survived a brutal attack by the Taliban and went on to become a global advocate for girls' education. Despite facing unimaginable adversity, Malala's unwavering courage and resilience enabled her to defy the odds and inspire millions around the world.

In essence, resilience is not merely a trait possessed by a select few but a skill that can be developed and strengthened through intentional effort and practice. By incorporating strategies such as mindfulness, cognitive-behavioral therapy, and gratitude journaling into our daily lives, we can cultivate resilience and empower ourselves to navigate life's challenges with grace and equanimity.

Summary

Chapter 1 of our narrative unfolds with a riveting account from childhood—a heart-stopping brush with danger that serves as a poignant reminder of the resilience and fortitude inherent within the human spirit. This pivotal event foreshadows a life trajectory defined by daring exploits and unwavering determination, where each challenge is met with a steadfast resolve and an unyielding spirit.

As a fervent sports enthusiast and natural leader, Michael embarks on a journey characterized by passion, dedication, and triumph. From the thrill of victory on the ice to the honor of leading a championship-winning team, his journey is a testament to the transformative power of perseverance and sheer determination.

Yet, life's journey is fraught with unexpected twists and turns, as demonstrated by the ill-fated decision to embark on a snowmobile ride amidst a blizzard. What ensues is a harrowing ordeal of survival, where the indomitable human spirit is pitted against the merciless forces of nature. Through sheer grit and raw determination, our protagonist navigates the treacherous terrain of pain and uncertainty, emerging victorious against overwhelming odds.

Recovery becomes a grueling uphill battle—a true test of character and resilience. With unwavering resolve, our narrator confronts the daunting specter of permanent injury, defying the limitations imposed by physical trauma with an unwavering determination. Through the transformative power of the mind and body, each step forward serves as a testament to the remarkable capacity for healing and renewal.

This chapter lays the foundation for a compelling narrative of courage and redemption, underscoring the enduring truth that even in the face of adversity, the human spirit remains unconquerable. It is a stirring testament to the resilience of the human spirit, a testament to the unyielding resolve to defy the odds and emerge stronger, braver, and more resilient than ever before.

Chapter 2

Goodbye Too Soon

*"In the end, it's not the years in your life that count.
It's the life in your years."*
~ **Abraham Lincoln**, 16th President of the United States, known for leading the country through the Civil War and abolishing slavery.

2

The Precipice of Change

Life's journey is a tapestry woven with threads of chance and destiny, where a single moment can alter the course of our existence in ways we never imagined. For me, that pivotal moment arrived like the sudden illumination of a dimly lit room—the discovery of the missing puzzle piece that completed the intricate mosaic of my life. It was a serendipitous encounter with Jen that forever changed the trajectory of my path, propelling me into a realm of love and possibility I never dared to dream of.

In the wake of my near-fatal accident, the gym transformed into more than just a place of physical rehabilitation—it became my sanctuary, a sacred space where I painstakingly pieced together the fragments of my shattered body, one grueling workout at a time. And it was within those hallowed walls that fate intervened, orchestrating a reunion that would alter the course of my life forever.

Jen, once a distant high school acquaintance, emerged from the shadows of memory as a radiant beacon of hope and healing. As our eyes met across the crowded gym floor, it was as though time stood still, and in that fleeting moment, I knew that my life would never be the same. The spark of recognition ignited a flame of connection—a connection that transcended the boundaries of time and space, binding our souls together in a dance of destiny.

Our love story unfolded with the breathtaking intensity of a wildfire, fueled by a shared passion for holistic wellness and a deep resonance of spirit. Like two puzzle pieces destined to fit seamlessly together, our hearts found solace and completion in each other's embrace. And as we embarked on this journey of love and partnership, it was clear that our union was not merely happenstance, but a divine orchestration of fate.

With each passing day, our bond grew stronger, our dreams intertwined like vines reaching for the sun. Together, we envisioned a future filled with love, laughter, and limitless possibility. And it was amidst this backdrop of shared dreams that the seeds of Life Yoga were planted—a vision born from the depths of our hearts, destined to flourish and bloom in the sanctuary of our shared home.

As the pages of our love story turned, whispers of uncertainty and foreboding danced on the edges of our consciousness, casting a faint shadow over the tapestry of our once-idyllic union. Unbeknownst to us, the winds of fate were poised to unleash a tempest that would rock the very foundation of our love, shaking us to our core and forcing us to confront the depths of our vulnerability.

In the quiet moments between whispered endearments and shared laughter, a subtle unease crept into the corners of our hearts—a silent harbinger of the trials yet to come. Little did we realize that amidst the gentle ebb and flow of our relationship lay a darkness that threatened to engulf us, leaving scars that would forever alter the landscape of our souls.

As we clung to each other in the face of uncertainty, the specter of tragedy loomed ever closer, its shadow stretching across the canvas of our shared dreams. And though we tried to outrun the storm, its relentless pursuit was inevitable, casting a pall over our once-bright future.

In the quiet moments of solitude, I caught fleeting glimpses of a future shrouded in sorrow, haunted by the specter of loss and grief. And though I tried to push these dark thoughts aside, a sense of impending doom lingered in the air, foretelling a fate that would forever change the course of our lives.

The Unthinkable Silence

Birthdays mark the passage of time, moments to pause and contemplate the journey traveled and the road yet to be ventured. For me, these annual celebrations were synonymous with shared camaraderie and boundless joy. However, the dawn of January 9, 2011, shattered that tradition with a silence so profound, it seemed to strip the air from our lungs.

Returning home, my heart brimming with anticipation for Jen's warm embrace, I was instead greeted by a chilling void—an abyss of emptiness that reverberated through the walls. The once-familiar couch, a sanctuary of shared laughter and quiet companionship, now bore the weight of her absence like a leaden cloak. It was in that haunting moment of realization that the truth crashed upon me like an avalanche—Jen had departed this world by her own hand, leaving behind a wake of unanswerable questions and unfathomable sorrow.

The crushing weight of her absence descended upon me, suffocating me with a grief so profound, it eclipsed any storm I had weathered before. How could she, the radiant beacon of light in my life, have succumbed to the darkness that now engulfed me? What demons had besieged her soul, driving her to the brink of irreparable despair? And how, amidst the labyrinth of anguish, could I navigate the tortuous path of grief without her steady hand to guide me?

These questions echoed relentlessly within the chambers of my mind, each one a serrated blade tearing at the fabric of my being. Yet amid the tempest of sorrow, a flicker of determination emerged—a resolve to unearth the truth behind Jen's tragic departure and to honor her memory by charting a course through the shadowy depths that lay ahead.

Standing at the precipice of this unfathomable loss, I understood that the journey ahead would test the very limits of my endurance and resilience, pushing me to confront emotions I had never imagined possible. But with each faltering step forward, guided by the dim but unwavering flame of hope that still burned within me, I pledged to persevere. Forging ahead through the darkness, I vowed to seek out the glimmering beacon of light that would ultimately guide me back to myself.

To those who have lost someone dear, know that you are not alone in your sorrow. In the midst of the darkest nights, may you find solace in the enduring light of hope and the unwavering strength of the human spirit. Though the road may be arduous and the burdens heavy, let us walk together, bound by the common thread of resilience, and emerge from the shadows, stronger and more whole than before.

Understanding Suicide

Suicide, a deeply intricate and devastating phenomenon, casts a long shadow over individuals and communities worldwide. It's a multifaceted issue rooted in a complex interplay of factors, encompassing mental health disorders, past traumas, substance abuse, and the weight of societal expectations. According to extensive research conducted by the World Health Organization (WHO), nearly 800,000 lives are lost to suicide each year, marking it as one of the leading causes of death globally.

The path to suicidal thoughts is often paved with layers of psychological and emotional trauma, leaving individuals feeling as though they are navigating an endless maze of despair. From the throes of untreated mental health conditions to the haunting echoes of past traumas, the burden of emotional pain can become overwhelmingly heavy. Studies have shown that individuals grappling with suicidal ideation often experience a profound sense of hopelessness, a feeling of being trapped in a cycle of anguish with no apparent escape route.

For those who find themselves or their loved ones ensnared in the grip of suicidal thoughts, seeking help is not just an option—it's an urgent imperative. The National Suicide Prevention Lifeline (1-800-273-TALK) stands as a beacon of hope, offering confidential support and resources for individuals teetering on the brink of crisis. Similarly, online platforms such as Suicide.org provide a wealth of information and guidance for those grappling with the aftermath of suicide, offering a lifeline in moments of profound darkness.

It's crucial to recognize that grappling with thoughts of suicide is not a sign of weakness, but rather a distress signal—a desperate cry for relief from unrelenting emotional pain. With the right support and intervention, individuals can navigate the tumultuous waters of despair and find their way back to a place of hope and healing. Research has shown that evidence-based treatments, such as therapy and medication, coupled with compassionate support from loved ones and mental health professionals, can significantly reduce the risk of suicide and pave the way for a brighter tomorrow.

To anyone wrestling with the weight of suicidal thoughts, know that you are not alone in your struggle. Your pain is valid, and there is hope for a better tomorrow. Reach out, lean on the support systems available, and remember that healing is possible. As you navigate the darkest corners of your mind, may you find solace in the knowledge that brighter days lie ahead, waiting to illuminate your path with renewed hope and resilience.

Understanding Post-Traumatic Stress Syndrome (PTSD)

Post-Traumatic Stress Disorder (PTSD) is a profound mental health condition that can arise in the aftermath of experiencing or witnessing a traumatic event. It's like an invisible scar, etched into the very fabric of one's being, leaving a trail of emotional wreckage in its wake. The symptoms of PTSD are as diverse as the individuals who experience them, ranging from debilitating flashbacks and haunting nightmares to overwhelming anxiety and intrusive thoughts that refuse to relent. Research indicates that PTSD affects approximately 7-8% of the population at some point in their lives, underscoring the pervasive nature of this silent torment.

The psychological and emotional toll of PTSD is profound, seeping into every corner of one's existence like an insidious fog. For those grappling with the aftermath of trauma, each day can feel like an uphill battle, a relentless struggle against the ghosts of the past that refuse to be silenced. The weight of PTSD can manifest in myriad ways, disrupting sleep, eroding relationships, and hijacking one's sense of safety and security in the world. Studies have shown that individuals with PTSD are at an increased risk of developing co-occurring mental health conditions, such as depression and substance abuse, further exacerbating their distress.

Navigating the labyrinth of PTSD often requires a multifaceted approach to treatment, one that addresses the complex interplay of psychological, emotional, and physiological factors at play. Therapy, particularly modalities like cognitive-behavioral therapy (CBT) and eye movement desensitization and reprocessing (EMDR), can provide individuals with the tools to confront and process their traumatic experiences, gradually reclaiming a sense of agency over their lives. Medication, such as antidepressants or anti-anxiety medications, may also be prescribed to alleviate symptoms and restore a semblance of balance to one's mental health.

In addition to professional intervention, the power of peer support and community cannot be understated in the journey towards healing from PTSD. Organizations like the National Center for PTSD serve as invaluable resources, offering a wealth of information and support for individuals and families navigating the complexities of this condition. Online platforms like PTSD United provide safe spaces for individuals to connect with others who share similar experiences, fostering a sense of belonging and solidarity in the face of adversity.

It's imperative to recognize that seeking help for PTSD is not a sign of weakness, but rather an act of courage and self-compassion. Healing from trauma takes time, patience, and unwavering dedication, but it is possible. To anyone grappling with the silent torment of PTSD, know that you are not alone in your struggle. Reach out, lean on your support network, and take the first step towards reclaiming your life from the shadows of the past. With resilience, perseverance, and the right support, brighter days lie ahead, waiting to embrace you with renewed hope and healing.

Cultivating Resilience:

Resilience is the beacon of light that guides us through the darkest of storms, the unwavering belief that even in the face of adversity, we possess the strength to rise again. It's not merely a trait bestowed upon the fortunate few, but rather a skill that can be cultivated and honed through intentional practice and perseverance. Research has shown that resilience is not a fixed quality but rather a dynamic process, shaped by our experiences, choices, and mindset.

Consider the humble oak tree, its roots firmly anchored in the earth, weathering countless storms and seasons. With each gust of wind and battering rain, it learns to bend without breaking, drawing upon the depth of its resilience to withstand the harshest of conditions. Similarly, as individuals, we possess an innate capacity for resilience, a wellspring of inner strength waiting to be tapped into.

In our daily lives, we encounter myriad challenges, both big and small, that serve as opportunities to flex our resilience muscles. From navigating a stressful work deadline to coping with the loss of a loved one, each trial presents a chance to cultivate resilience. It's in the moments of adversity that we discover our true capacity for growth and transformation, as we learn to adapt, evolve, and emerge stronger than before.

Practicing mindfulness is one powerful tool in our resilience-building arsenal, offering a pathway to cultivate inner peace and emotional stability amidst life's tumultuous currents. By tuning into the present moment with curiosity and compassion, we develop a greater sense of self-awareness and emotional regulation, empowering us to navigate challenges with grace and resilience.

Engaging in self-care activities is another vital aspect of resilience-building, as it allows us to replenish our physical, emotional, and mental reserves. Whether it's taking a leisurely stroll in nature, indulging in a creative hobby, or simply prioritizing adequate rest, self-care acts as a lifeline in times of stress, helping us recharge and rejuvenate our spirits.

Furthermore, fostering strong social connections serves as a cornerstone of resilience, providing us with a robust support network to lean on during difficult times. By nurturing meaningful relationships built on trust, empathy, and reciprocity, we create a sense of belonging and solidarity that bolsters our resilience in the face of adversity.

In essence, resilience is not about avoiding stress or hardship but rather about embracing life's challenges with courage, fortitude, and optimism. It's about recognizing our innate capacity for growth and transformation, even in the midst of adversity. So, to anyone grappling with life's trials and tribulations, remember that within you lies the power to overcome, to thrive, and to emerge stronger than ever before. Cultivate resilience, nurture it like the precious seed it is, and watch as it blossoms into a beacon of hope and strength in your life's journey.

Shifting Perspective

"When you change the way you look at things, the things you look at change."
— **Wayne Dyer**

Perspective is the lens through which we view the world, shaping our perceptions, decisions, and ultimately, our reality. It's the unique vantage point from which we interpret life's experiences, colored by our beliefs, values, and past experiences. Yet, despite its subjectivity, perspective holds immense power in influencing our responses to life's challenges and shaping our overall well-being.

At its core, perspective encompasses not only what we see, but also how we interpret and make meaning of what we see. It's the difference between viewing a setback as a roadblock or as an opportunity for growth, between seeing adversity as a burden or as a chance to cultivate resilience. Research has shown that adopting a growth mindset, which emphasizes learning and development, can lead to greater resilience and psychological well-being. By reframing negative experiences as opportunities for growth and learning, individuals can shift their perspective from one of defeat to one of empowerment.

However, mastering perspective is no easy feat. Our minds are inherently predisposed to biases, influenced by a myriad of factors ranging from cultural upbringing to cognitive shortcuts. As such, our perspective is often filtered through the lens of these biases, leading to distorted perceptions and flawed decision-making. The quote "strong opinions, loosely held" encapsulates the essence of perspective, reminding us to hold our beliefs with conviction while remaining open to new information and alternative viewpoints.

To improve our skill of perspective, it's essential to cultivate mindfulness and self-awareness. By becoming attuned to our thought patterns and biases, we can begin to challenge and reframe negative interpretations, allowing for greater flexibility and openness in our perspective. Practicing gratitude offers another pathway to shifting perspective, inviting us to focus on the positives in our lives and fostering a sense of abundance and appreciation.

Real-life examples abound of how perspective can shape our experiences. Consider the individual who loses their job and views it as a devastating blow to their self-worth, versus the one who sees it as an opportunity to pursue a new career path or embark on a journey of self-discovery. Or the person who encounters a rude stranger and interprets it as a personal attack, versus the one who chooses to respond with compassion and understanding, recognizing that the other person may be struggling with their own challenges.

Ultimately, cultivating a growth-oriented perspective is a lifelong journey, one that requires patience, self-reflection, and a willingness to embrace discomfort. By recognizing the power of perspective in shaping our reality, and actively working to expand our view of the world, we can unlock new possibilities for growth, resilience, and fulfillment in our lives. So, I encourage you to approach each day with curiosity and openness, knowing that by shifting your perspective, you have the power to transform challenges into opportunities and adversity into growth.

Nurturing a Positive Mindset

A positive mindset is not merely a luxury but a necessity for navigating life's challenges with grace and resilience. Countless studies have shown the profound impact of positive thinking on mental and emotional well-being. When we embrace positivity, we not only enhance our ability to bounce back from adversity but also reduce the harmful effects of stress on our minds and body.

Research has demonstrated that positive thinking can lead to a host of physiological benefits, including reduced levels of cortisol, the stress hormone, and increased production of endorphins, the body's natural painkillers. By maintaining a positive outlook, individuals can effectively mitigate the negative impact of stress on their health, promoting overall well-being and longevity.

One study conducted by the University of California, Berkeley, found that individuals who regularly engaged in positive thinking practices, such as gratitude journaling and visualization, exhibited lower levels of inflammatory markers associated with chronic stress. These findings underscore the profound influence of positive thinking on our physiological responses to stress, highlighting its role in promoting resilience and protecting against the detrimental effects of stress-related illness.

So, how can we cultivate a more positive mindset in our daily lives? One powerful tool is mindfulness, which involves paying attention to the present moment without judgment. By practicing mindfulness meditation or simply engaging in mindful activities such as deep breathing or mindful eating, we can train our minds to focus on the here and now, fostering a sense of peace and contentment.

Setting realistic goals is another effective strategy for nurturing positivity. By setting achievable objectives and celebrating our progress along the way, we can cultivate a sense of accomplishment and optimism. Surrounding ourselves with supportive people who uplift and encourage us can also bolster our positive outlook, providing a sense of connection and belonging that fuels our resilience in the face of adversity.

Ultimately, positivity is a choice—a conscious decision to focus on the good in life and approach challenges with optimism and resilience. By embracing positivity as a way of life, we not only create a brighter, more fulfilling future for ourselves but also inspire those around us to do the same. So, I encourage you to harness the power of positive thinking, knowing that by doing so, you can transform adversity into opportunity and cultivate a life filled with joy, purpose, and resilience.

Once you have started to understand your current mindset, you can begin to transform it by creating new and empowering belief statements, also known as affirmations. The key is creating statements that work with your subconscious mind and not against it. If you are saying something on a conscious level that you have never experienced, your mind will more than likely call bullshit on you. But there is a loophole. Your subconscious does not know the difference between what is real and what is vividly imagined. If you change your statements from "I am depressed" to "I am in the process of healing" your subconscious mind doesn't argue that because you are in the process of healing.

~ **Brenda Johnston**
Subconscious Mindset Strategist & Energy Mentor

The Spiral

The aftermath of Jen's loss plunged me into a darkness so profound, it felt like being swallowed whole by an unfathomable abyss. The pain of her absence, a relentless ache that tore at my heart, seemed insurmountable, eclipsing even the most agonizing physical traumas I had ever endured. Each day was a battle against the suffocating weight of despair, as I struggled to find meaning in a world that suddenly seemed devoid of light.

In the midst of this overwhelming darkness, I found myself grappling with an old adversary—painkillers. What had once been a temporary refuge from physical agony now beckoned to me as a sinister escape from the unbearable reality of Jen's absence. The allure of numbness, of temporary relief from the searing pain of grief, proved dangerously seductive, pulling me into a downward spiral of addiction and despair.

As the grip of addiction tightened its hold on me, I felt myself slipping further into the abyss, losing sight of any semblance of hope or redemption. It was a treacherous path, fraught with danger and despair, where each step seemed to lead me deeper into the darkness. Yet, even in my darkest hour, there were those who refused to let me drown.

Family, friends, and loved ones became my lifeline, offering unwavering support and compassion as I battled the demons within. Their presence, a beacon of light in the darkness, reminded me that I was not alone in my struggle—that there were people who cared for me, who believed in my ability to overcome adversity.

With their encouragement and support, I began to find the strength to confront my addiction head-on, to seek help and treatment for the demons that threatened to consume me. It was a journey fraught with setbacks and challenges, but with each step forward, I felt myself inching closer to the light.

The road to recovery was long and arduous, marked by moments of triumph and moments of despair. But through it all, I clung to the glimmer of hope that burned within me, a beacon guiding me through the darkest of nights. And though the journey was far from easy, I emerged on the other side stronger and more resilient than I ever thought possible.

In the end, it was the love and support of those who refused to give up on me that carried me through the darkest chapters of my life. Their unwavering faith in my ability to overcome adversity became my guiding light, illuminating the path to redemption and renewal. And though the scars of my past may never fully fade, they serve as a testament to the strength and resilience that lie within us all, waiting to be unleashed in the face of adversity.

From Despair to Hope

Entangled in the unforgiving clutches of addiction, I found myself teetering on the brink of losing everything I held dear. The looming threat of legal consequences, poised to unravel the foundation of my life's work, cast a shadow so dark it threatened to suffocate any lingering hope within me. It was as if my very existence hung in the balance, caught between the jaws of despair and the fleeting glimmer of redemption.

But amidst the wreckage of my shattered dreams, a beacon of unexpected grace illuminated the hallowed halls of the courtroom. The granting of an absolute discharge, accompanied by the weighty admonition of a final warning, marked a pivotal juncture in my tumultuous journey—a moment of reckoning, where the pendulum swung between condemnation and clemency. It was a second chance at redemption, a lifeline thrown to me in the midst of the tempest, and I seized it with a fervor born of desperation and determination.

This chapter of my life served as a poignant testament to the delicate balance between fragility and resilience, the capricious dance of fate that weaves its threads through the tapestry of our existence. In the wake of Jen's absence, I embarked on a soul-stirring odyssey of self-discovery—a pilgrimage into the depths of my own sorrow and longing, in search of the flickering embers of renewal and rebirth.

It was a journey that demanded courage and fortitude, a willingness to confront the darkest recesses of my being and emerge transformed on the other side. For I soon realized that healing is not merely about mending the wounds of the past, but about embracing the crucible of adversity as a catalyst for metamorphosis. It is about surrendering to the alchemy of grief and loss, allowing it to sculpt us into beings of greater depth and resilience than we ever thought possible.

Armed with resolve and resilience as my guiding lights, I navigated the turbulent waters of grief with an unwavering spirit. Each trial and tribulation became a crucible in which my character was forged, each setback a stepping stone on the path to redemption. And though battered and bruised by the storms of life, I emerged from the crucible of despair not as a shattered remnant of my former self, but as a phoenix rising from the ashes—renewed, revitalized, and unbroken.

Navigating the Wake of Loss

Jen's departure from this world cast a profound and enduring shadow over every facet of my existence—a shadow that stretched across the landscape of my life, obscuring the once-vibrant hues with the somber tones of grief and loss. It was a relentless reminder of the ephemeral nature of life itself, and the devastating aftermath of emotional trauma that reverberates long after the initial shock has faded into memory.

As I navigated the labyrinthine depths of grief, Life Yoga—a sanctuary of shared dreams and aspirations between Jen and me—passed into the capable hands of a trusted friend. Their stewardship of our collective vision brought a measure of solace, knowing that the legacy of our shared passion would endure, carried forth with grace and dignity in the wake of our absence. Yet, for me, the path forward remained obscured by the looming specter of uncertainty—a path strewn with the shattered remnants of dreams unfulfilled and promises left unkept.

In the wake of Jen's absence, each fleeting relationship became a fleeting beacon of hope—a tenuous lifeline cast adrift in the stormy seas of grief. Yet, try as I might to seek solace in the arms of transient companionship, the void left by Jen's departure remained unyielding, a silent abyss that threatened to engulf me whole. With each passing day, the chasm within me only seemed to deepen, echoing the silent scream of grief that reverberated within the caverns of my soul—a haunting refrain that served as a constant reminder of the irrevocable loss that had befallen me.

But even amidst the suffocating grip of despair, there lingered a glimmer of hope—a faint ember that refused to be extinguished. It was a testament to the resilience of the human spirit, a fragile flame that flickered defiantly against the encroaching darkness. And though the path ahead remained fraught with uncertainty and sorrow, I clung to that flickering light with a tenacity born of desperation and determination, knowing that even in the darkest of nights, there exists the possibility of dawn.

The Relentless Grip of Addiction

Sobriety, a journey fraught with peril, became a precarious tightrope walk over the yawning abyss of relapse—a delicate dance between the promise of healing and the ever-present specter of temptation. Painkillers, once a fleeting respite from the relentless grip of physical agony, now beckoned to me with a seductive allure, whispering promises of temporary relief from the ceaseless onslaught of emotional turmoil that threatened to engulf me.

Each pill swallowed was a descent into the depths of addiction—a descent fueled by the haunting memory of Jen's absence, which loomed large like a shadow cast across the landscape of my existence.

The journey of sobriety, fraught with its own formidable challenges, demanded a level of resilience and resolve that I never knew I possessed. It required a constant vigilance, a steadfast determination to resist the siren's call of addiction even as it whispered sweet promises of escape. Yet, with each passing day, the struggle became more arduous, the weight of Jen's absence pressing down upon me like a leaden cloak, suffocating me with its relentless grip.

And yet, amidst the darkness, there remained a glimmer of hope—a fragile ember that refused to be extinguished. It was a reminder that even in the depths of despair, there existed the possibility of redemption, of reclaiming a life untethered by the chains of addiction. With each faltering step along the path to sobriety, I clung to that flickering light with a fierce determination, knowing that it was the only beacon that could guide me back from the brink of oblivion.

Addiction: Navigating the Complexities of Substance Abuse

Addiction is a complex and pervasive issue that affects millions of individuals worldwide, including many who have experienced trauma and loss. Understanding the nature of addiction is crucial for those grappling with its effects, as well as for their loved ones and support networks.

Prevalence of Addiction

In North America, addiction manifests in various forms, with substance abuse being one of the most prevalent types. According to recent studies, the top five main addictions in North America include alcohol, tobacco, opioids, stimulants, and cannabis. These addictions collectively affect millions of individuals, leading to significant health, social, and economic consequences.

Research indicates that substance abuse is a widespread issue, with approximately 21 million Americans struggling with at least one addiction. Moreover, the National Institute on Drug Abuse (NIDA) reports that substance abuse costs the United States more than $740 billion annually in healthcare, crime-related expenses, and lost productivity.

Impact on the Brain

Addiction is not merely a matter of personal choice or willpower; it is a complex neurobiological disorder that affects the brain's functioning. When individuals engage in addictive behaviors, such as substance abuse, their brains undergo profound changes that alter their thoughts, feelings, and behaviors.

Studies have shown that addiction primarily affects the brain's reward system, hijacking its normal functioning and leading to compulsive drug-seeking and use. The neurotransmitter dopamine, often referred to as the "pleasure chemical," plays a central role in this process, reinforcing behaviors associated with substance abuse and creating a cycle of craving and reward.

Additionally, addiction impacts other brain regions responsible for decision-making, impulse control, and emotional regulation, further exacerbating addictive behaviors. Over time, these changes can lead to tolerance, dependence, and withdrawal symptoms, making it increasingly difficult for individuals to quit using substances.

The Link to Emotional Trauma and Grief

For many individuals, addiction is intertwined with experiences of emotional trauma and grief, as was the case for me after losing Jen. Trauma and loss can trigger intense emotional pain and distress, driving individuals to seek solace in substances as a means of coping. Research suggests that individuals who have experienced trauma are more susceptible to developing addiction as a maladaptive coping mechanism.

Moreover, unresolved grief and trauma can exacerbate addictive behaviors, creating a vicious cycle of substance abuse and emotional distress. In my own journey, the profound sense of loss and emptiness left by Jen's suicide propelled me into a downward spiral of addiction, as I sought to numb the pain and escape the overwhelming grief.

Understanding addiction requires a multifaceted approach that addresses its biological, psychological, and social dimensions. By recognizing addiction as a complex neurobiological disorder with deep roots in emotional trauma and grief, we can begin to dismantle the stigma surrounding it and offer more compassionate and effective support to those in need.

If you or someone you know is struggling with addiction, know that you are not alone. Reach out for help, whether it's through support groups, therapy, or rehabilitation programs. Recovery is possible, and with the right support and resources, you can reclaim your life and embark on a journey of healing and renewal.

Understanding and Forgiveness

Understanding and coming to terms with suicide is akin to navigating through a dense fog – the path ahead is obscured, and the weight of guilt and confusion weighs heavy on the heart. Yet, as time unfolds, clarity emerges, revealing the hidden complexities and silent struggles that often precede such tragic events.

Suicide shrouds itself in secrecy, veiling its presence from even the keenest observers. Jen's past traumas, concealed beneath a veneer of calm, served as the silent undercurrents pulling her into the depths of despair. Her journey into yoga, though a testament to her resilience, belied the storm raging within – a storm I failed to recognize until it was too late. Through introspection and empathy, I came to understand that suicide's cloak is woven with threads of anguish and isolation, invisible to all but those who bear its burden.

Jen's story serves as a poignant reminder of the critical role we play in each other's lives. By reaching out, checking in, and offering support, we can extend a lifeline to those silently battling their inner demons. The signs may be subtle, the cries for help whispered, but by listening closely and loving fiercely, we can break through the silence and offer hope in the face of despair. In honoring Jen's memory, we pledge to be vigilant guardians of each other's well-being, recognizing that our actions – no matter how small – can make a world of difference to someone in need.

Embracing Compassion and Forgiveness

Amidst the wreckage of grief and guilt, forgiveness emerges as a beacon of light, illuminating the path forward. Forgiveness is not about absolving blame or forgetting the pain; rather, it is a profound act of self-compassion and understanding. By extending forgiveness to ourselves and others, we release the burdens of resentment and regret, opening our hearts to healing and transformation. Through Jen's story, I learned that forgiveness is not a one-time gesture but a journey of acceptance and grace, paving the way for healing and redemption.

As we journey through the complexities of suicide and loss, may we find solace in the power of understanding and forgiveness. May Jen's story serve as a catalyst for compassion and empathy, inspiring us to reach out, listen deeply, and love unconditionally. In the quiet moments of reflection, may we honor the silent struggles and unspoken cries for help, and may our collective efforts pave the way for a brighter, more compassionate future.

The Importance of Forgiveness

Forgiveness is a deeply personal and complex process that holds the key to healing emotional wounds and restoring inner peace. Research in psychology and neuroscience has shed light on the profound effects of forgiveness on our mental and physical well-being. Studies have shown that practicing forgiveness can lead to reduced stress, improved mood, and enhanced overall health.

Psychological Reasons for Forgiveness

Forgiveness is not about condoning or excusing harmful behavior; rather, it is a conscious decision to release resentment and let go of the emotional burden carried from past hurts. Psychologically, forgiveness liberates us from the grip of bitterness and anger, allowing us to reclaim our power and autonomy. By reframing our perspective and embracing empathy, we can cultivate compassion and understanding for ourselves and others.

Neurobiological Effects of Forgiveness

Neuroscience research has revealed that forgiveness has tangible effects on the brain, reshaping neural pathways associated with negative emotions and fostering a sense of inner peace. Forgiveness activates brain regions involved in empathy, compassion, and reward processing, leading to feelings of connection and emotional well-being.

Tools for Practicing Forgiveness

Forgiveness is a skill that can be cultivated through intentional practice and self-reflection. One effective tool for practicing forgiveness is the "fourfold path" model, which involves acknowledging the hurt, fostering empathy, making a decision to forgive, and letting go of resentment. Additionally, mindfulness meditation and journaling can help individuals explore their emotions and cultivate a sense of forgiveness.

Forgiveness emerged as a guiding light on my journey of healing and redemption. Through understanding and compassion, I was able to release the weight of resentment and embrace forgiveness as a pathway to inner peace. As you navigate your own journey of healing from trauma and loss, may you find solace in the transformative power of forgiveness, and may Jen's story serve as a beacon of hope for those in search of light amidst the darkness of grief.

Summary

Chapter 2 delves into the depths of grief as I grapple with the sudden and devastating loss of Jen, my partner in life and business. The once-familiar sanctuary of the gym transforms into a haunting reminder of her absence, a space where memories of her laughter and presence linger like ghosts. Despite the daily responsibilities of managing Life Yoga, the studio we built together, Jen's absence is a constant ache, a bittersweet reminder of the vibrant spirit she brought to our shared dreams.

As I navigate the turbulent waters of grief, my personal life becomes a reflection of the inner turmoil I face. Attempting to fill the void left by Jen proves to be an impossible task, leading to a series of unfulfilled relationships and a sense of emptiness that refuses to dissipate. Sobriety becomes a precarious tightrope walk, with painkillers offering a temporary reprieve from the overwhelming pain of loss but ultimately dragging me deeper into the clutches of addiction.

Throughout this chapter, I confront the complex emotions surrounding suicide, grappling with feelings of self-blame and the haunting question of missed signs. Jen's untold struggles with a traumatic past shed light on the silent battles many face behind closed doors. Her dedication to yoga, once seen as a beacon of healing, reveals deeper wounds hidden beneath a facade of serenity. This chapter serves as a raw testament to the importance of vigilance and compassion in the face of hidden suffering, emphasizing the power of reaching out and the necessity of honest communication in the healing process.

Despite the darkness that envelops me, there remains a glimmer of hope—a recognition that even in the depths of despair, there is the potential for growth and renewal. Through vulnerability and openness, I begin to navigate the winding path of healing, embracing the lessons learned from Jen's tragic passing and committing to a future marked by resilience, understanding, and compassion. As I continue to journey through the aftermath of loss, I am reminded of the transformative power of love and the enduring strength of the human spirit to rise from the ashes of tragedy.

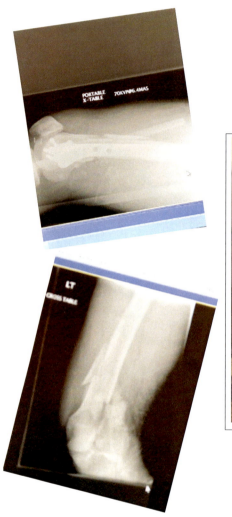
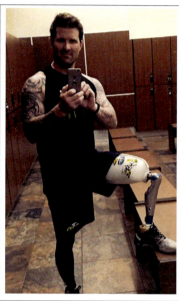

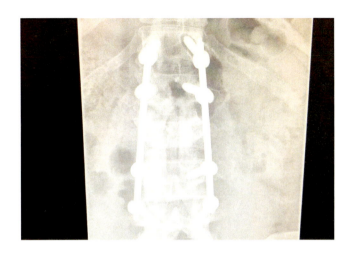

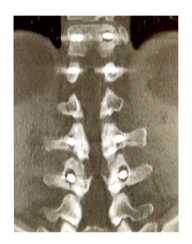

Untapped 60

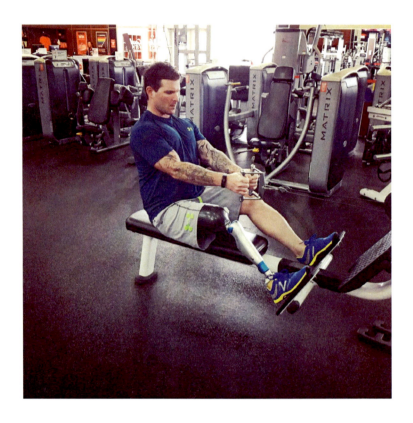

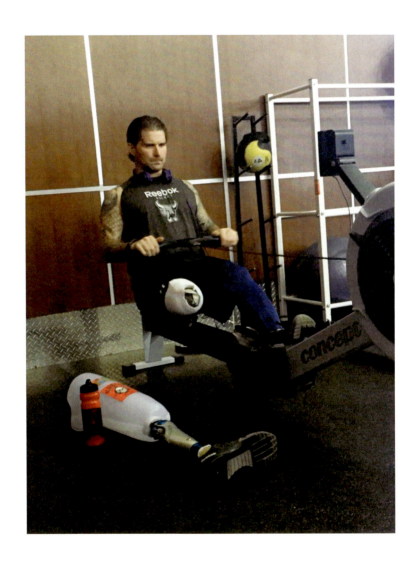

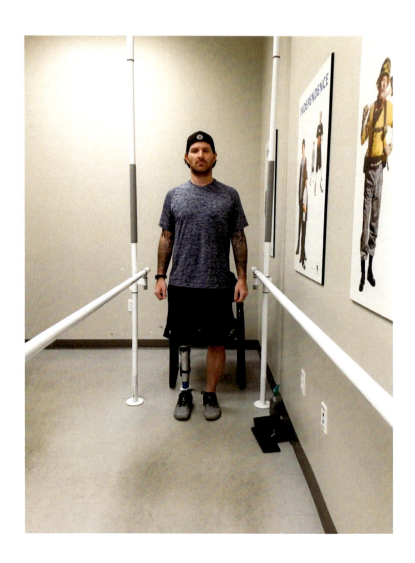

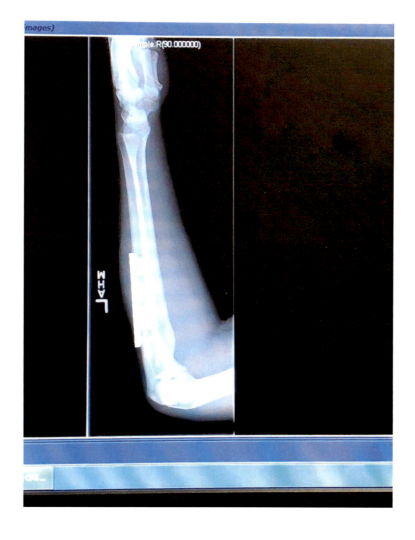

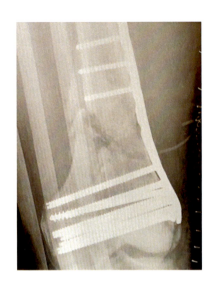

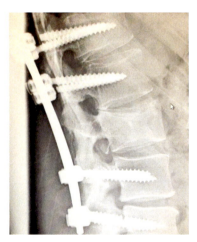

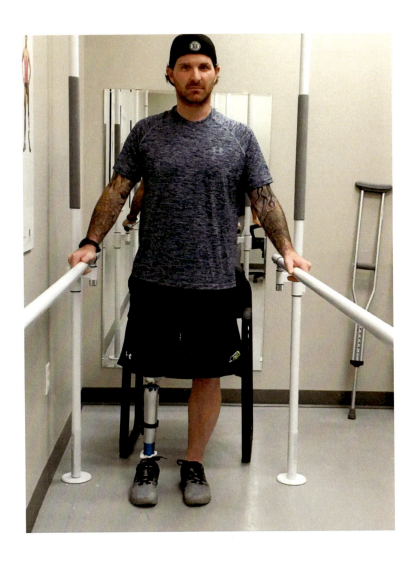

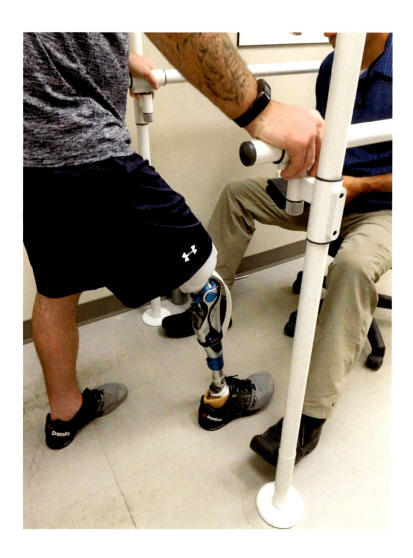

www.untapped60.com

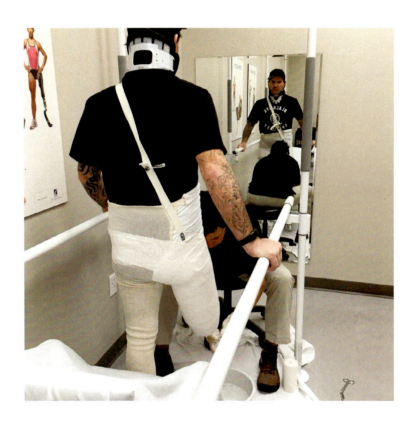

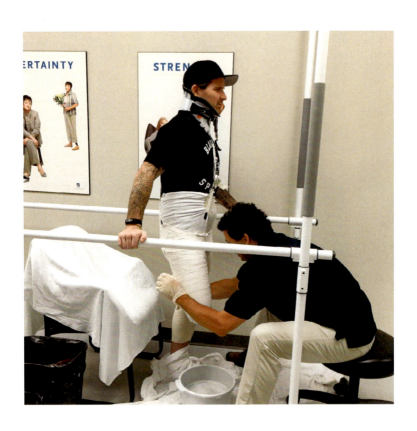

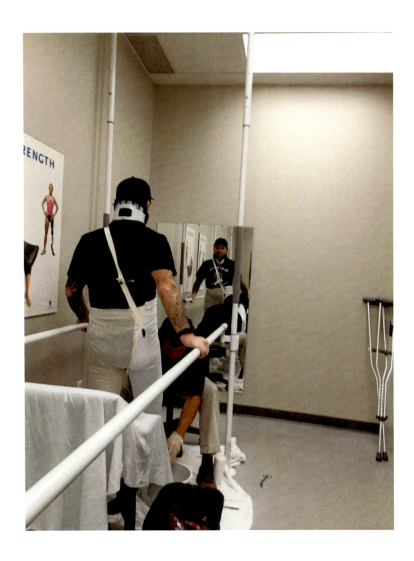

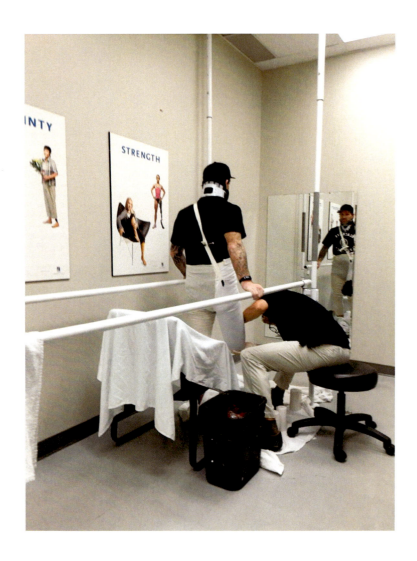

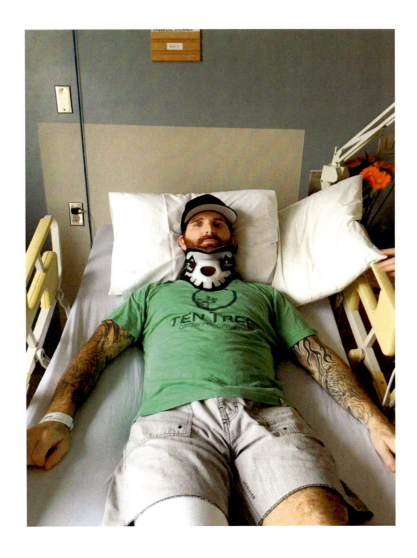

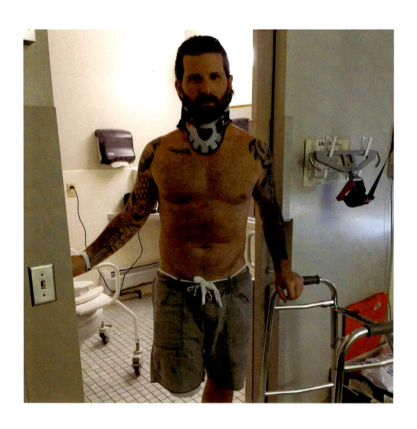

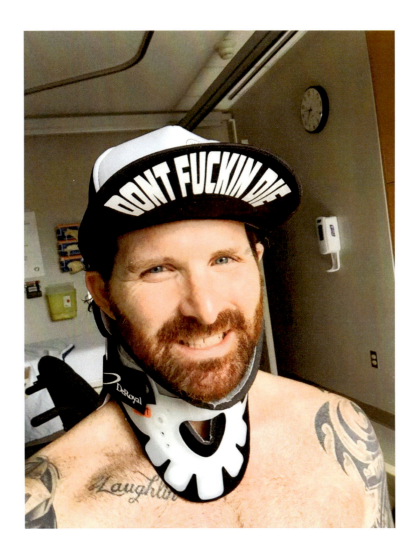

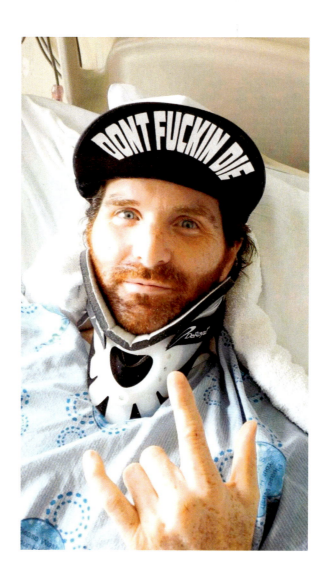

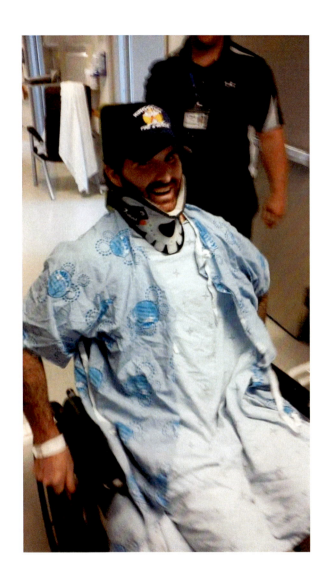

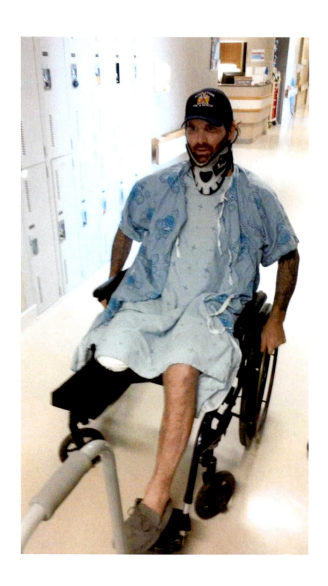

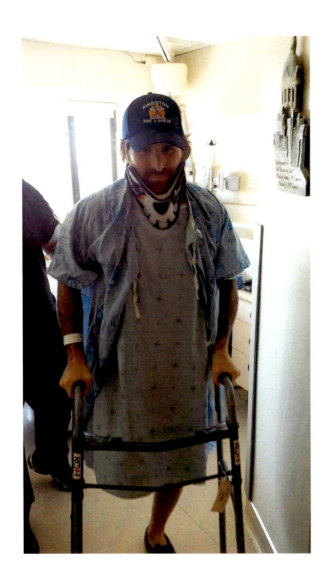

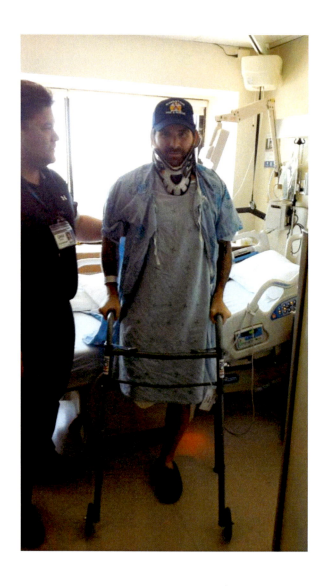

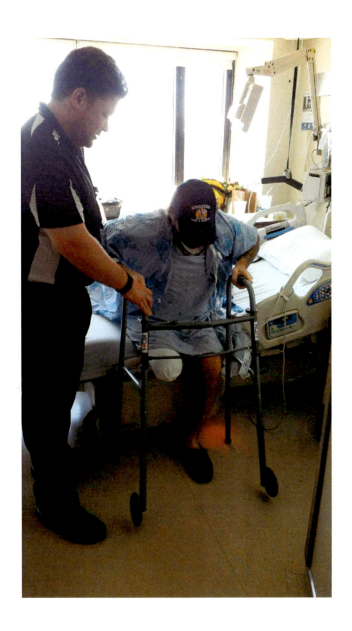

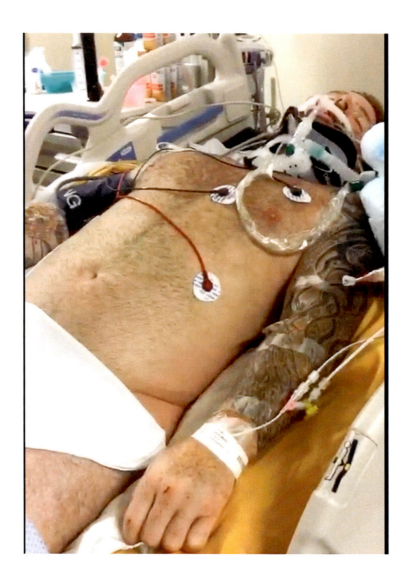

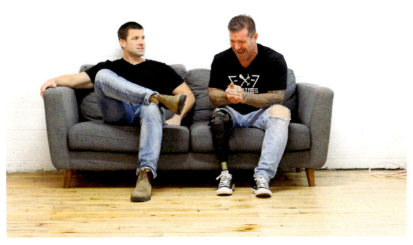

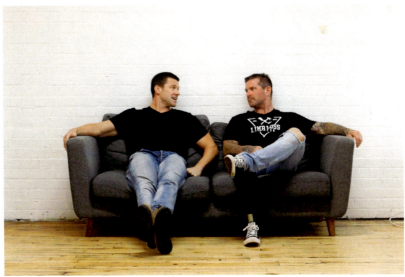

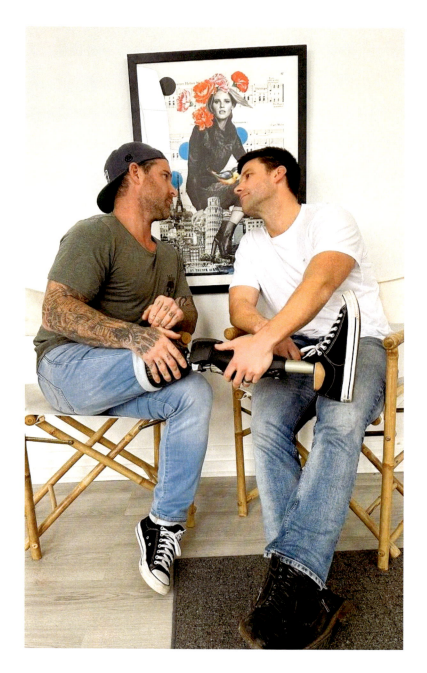

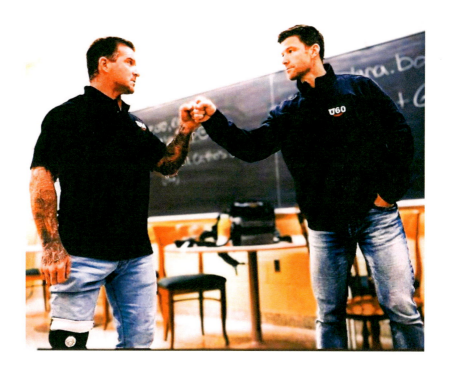

Chapter 3

Broken, Mended, Unstoppable

*"I am not afraid of storms
for I am learning how to sail my ship."*
~ **Louisa May Alcott**, celebrated author of *Little Women*, who was an abolitionist and feminist.

3

A Rider's Heartbeat

Immersed in the serene landscape of Joyceville, Ontario, Canada, my childhood unfolded against the backdrop of sprawling fields and the whisper of the wind through the trees. Yet, amidst this idyllic setting, my heartbeat to the rhythm of something more—the exhilarating pulse of engines and the aroma of motor oil that permeated the air. It was here, amid the rustic charm of our farm, that my love affair with motorcycles was kindled, igniting a passion that would shape the course of my life.

From the tender age when my legs first found solid ground, I was drawn like a magnet to anything that bore wheels and an engine. Whether it was the thrill of bounding across rugged terrain atop an ATV or the camaraderie of helping my father navigate the fields on his trusty tractor, I found solace and excitement in the embrace of horsepower and steel.

But beyond the rush of adrenaline and the allure of speed, motorcycles held a deeper significance for me. They were not merely machines; they were companions, steadfast and true, ready to whisk me away on exhilarating adventures at a moment's notice. Each ride became an odyssey—a voyage of liberation that offered respite from the monotony of everyday life.

The day I came of age to acquire my motorcycle license felt like an ascension to newfound freedom—a pivotal moment that marked the beginning of a lifelong journey. It was as though I had earned my wings, poised to soar into the boundless expanse of possibility that lay ahead.

By the time 2016 arrived, riding had become second nature to me. The rumble of the engine beneath me resonated like a reassuring heartbeat, a symphony of power that harmonized seamlessly with my own pulse. With every twist of the throttle and every lean into a curve, I felt a profound sense of connection—a fusion of man and machine, united in a dance of precision and exhilaration.

Little did I know that this very passion, which had brought me immeasurable joy and freedom, would soon become the catalyst for the most tumultuous chapter of my life. But for now, as I traversed the winding roads, the wind whipping through my hair and the sun casting its golden glow upon me, I felt invincible—a lone adventurer forging ahead into the unknown, brimming with anticipation for the adventures that awaited beyond the horizon.

Collision Course

One afternoon, as familiar with my bike as with the back of my hand, I embarked on my usual ride through the winding roads near Loughborough Lake. The sun hung lazily in the sky, casting long shadows across the asphalt as if warning of the impending danger ahead. The air was thick with the scent of pine and the promise of adventure, but little did I know, this ride would be unlike any other.

As I rounded a particularly sharp curve, my senses on high alert, a sudden movement caught my eye—a flash of brown fur darting across the road. In the blink of an eye, a deer materialized before me, its panicked eyes meeting mine in a moment of silent understanding. Time seemed to slow to a crawl as our fates collided in a heartbeat.

The impact was as sudden and jarring as a lightning strike, throwing my bike and me into a frantic wobble. It felt like being caught in a whirlwind, a chaotic dance with fate that left me teetering on the brink of disaster. Instinct and muscle memory battled against the forces of gravity and momentum, each twist and turn of the road a test of skill and survival.

In that split second, as the world spun wildly around me, I clung to the handlebars with a desperate determination, my heart pounding in my chest like a drumbeat of defiance. Every fiber of my being screamed at me to keep going, to fight against the inevitable pull of gravity and fate. But as the road twisted sharply ahead, reality crashed over me like a tidal wave, forcing me to confront the harsh truth—I was no match for the laws of physics and the merciless forces of nature.

As the bike careened towards the unforgiving pavement, my mind raced with a flurry of questions.

How had it come to this? What had I done to deserve such a cruel twist of fate? And most importantly, would I ever make it out of this alive?

But amidst the chaos and uncertainty, one thing became abundantly clear—I had to act, and I had to act fast. With every ounce of strength and determination I could muster, I braced myself for the inevitable impact, knowing that the outcome would shape the course of my life in ways I could never have imagined.

The World Upside Down

In the split second that followed the collision with the deer, my world turned upside down—quite literally. As my bike's foot peg grazed the pavement in a desperate attempt to navigate the treacherous corner, it felt as though time itself had slowed to a crawl, each passing second stretching out like taffy pulled to its limit. The familiar rumble of the engine was drowned out by the deafening roar of adrenaline coursing through my veins, and for a moment, all I could hear was the frantic thud of my heart in my ears.

But fate, it seemed, had other plans. With a sickening lurch, the bike's back tire found the gravel shoulder, and suddenly, we were skidding out of control. The world around me blurred into a chaotic whirlwind of motion, colors blending together like a watercolor painting left out in the rain. It was as if time had fractured, each fragment of reality spinning away into the abyss.

In that heart-stopping moment, as the laws of physics asserted their merciless dominance over my fate, I found myself confronted with a stark realization—the fragility of life, the fleeting nature of existence. It was a sobering revelation, one that pierced through the haze of fear and uncertainty like a beacon of truth in the darkness.

As the bike careened towards the unforgiving ground, my mind raced with a flurry of thoughts and emotions. Memories flashed before my eyes like scenes from a movie reel, each one a poignant reminder of the life I had lived and the people I held dear. In that moment of clarity, I found myself grappling with existential questions that had long remained unanswered—had I lived a life worth remembering? Had I made a difference in the world? And most importantly, would I ever get the chance to say goodbye to those I loved?

As the world spun wildly around me, I braced for impact, my body tensing instinctively in preparation for the inevitable collision. And in that moment of uncertainty, amidst the chaos and turmoil, I uttered a silent prayer—a plea for protection, for redemption, for a second chance at life. It was a desperate cry into the void, a final testament to the resilience of the human spirit in the face of overwhelming adversity.

Little did I know that this moment would mark the beginning of a journey that would test me in ways I could never have imagined, a journey that would ultimately redefine the very essence of my being. But for now, as I hurtled towards the ground with a velocity that seemed to defy comprehension, all I could do was hold on tight and pray for a miracle.

Ground Impact

The collision unleashed an earth-shattering symphony of destruction—a chorus of metal twisting and bones snapping In the split second before impact, time seemed to slow to a crawl, each heartbeat echoing like a drumbeat in my ears. The air crackled with tension, thick with the scent of burning rubber and the taste of impending doom.

As the bike careened off the road and into the unforgiving embrace of the ditch, I was thrown into a whirlwind of chaos and confusion. The world spun around me in a dizzying blur, colors bleeding together in a kaleidoscope of pain and fear. In those fleeting moments, a flood of thoughts and emotions surged through my mind like a raging river, threatening to overwhelm me.

Amidst the chaos, I found myself grappling with the stark reality of my mortality. More questions raced through my mind, unbidden and unstoppable. Had I lived a life of purpose and meaning? Would anyone remember me when I was gone? And most haunting of all, would my loved ones ever forgive me for leaving them behind?

The impact itself was a brutal assault on my senses—a visceral shock that reverberated through every fiber of my being. I felt the searing heat of the bike's metal against my skin, branding me with its fiery touch like a cruel reminder of my own mortality. The pain was blinding, excruciating, threatening to consume me whole.

But amidst the agony, amidst the chaos and confusion, a sense of clarity emerged—a final moment of lucidity in the face of impending oblivion. And in that moment, I found myself uttering a silent prayer—a plea for forgiveness, for redemption, for a chance to make things right. It was a desperate cry into the void, a final farewell to a world that was slipping away from me with every passing second.

As the darkness closed in around me, as the world faded into oblivion, I found solace in the knowledge that I had loved and been loved in return. And with my last breath, with my final whisper into the void, I uttered a single word—a word that echoed through the depths of my soul and beyond.

"Goodbye."

Self-Rescue

The world around me blurred into a haze of agony and disbelief as I glanced down, my eyes widening in horror at the sight below. My [good] leg, once a sturdy pillar of support, now hung grotesquely from my body, shattered and mangled like a broken branch dangling from a tree. The pain, searing and relentless, threatened to engulf me in a tidal wave of despair, but amidst the chaos, a primal instinct took hold—a survival instinct honed through years of training and adversity.

With trembling hands and a heart pounding in my chest, I sprang into action, the adrenaline coursing through my veins drowning out the screams of agony echoing in my mind. Ignoring the protests of my fractured body, I fumbled for my belt, the metal buckle a lifeline in the chaos. With a desperate urgency born of desperation, I fashioned a makeshift tourniquet, cinching it tight around my mangled limb, the pressure sending waves of pain shooting through my body but offering a fleeting sense of relief in the face of impending disaster.

As I struggled to maintain consciousness amidst the haze of pain and shock, a sense of surreal clarity washed over me. With my hands slick with blood and my vision swimming, I reached for my phone, fingers trembling as they dialed the familiar number of the fire dispatch. Each ring seemed to stretch into eternity, the silence of the line deafening in its intensity. And then, a voice—an anchor in the storm—answered on the other end, grounding me in the midst of chaos.

In that moment, as I clung to the precipice between life and death, a torrent of emotions threatened to overwhelm me. Fear, anger, despair—they swirled together in a whirlwind of confusion and disbelief, each one vying for dominance in the tempest raging within. But, once again, amidst the chaos, that same flicker of hope burned bright—a stubborn refusal to surrender to the darkness closing in around me.

As I awaited the arrival of help, a sense of determination surged through me—a fierce resolve to defy the odds and fight for survival against all odds. With each labored breath, with each beat of my battered heart, I refused to give in to the despair threatening to consume me. For in that moment, amidst the wreckage of my shattered body, I found a strength I never knew I possessed—a strength forged in the crucible of adversity and tempered by the fires of resilience.

And so, as I clung to life by the slimmest of threads, I made a silent vow—a promise to myself and to those I loved. A promise to endure, to overcome, to rise from the ashes of tragedy stronger and more determined than ever before. For in the face of unspeakable pain and unimaginable loss, there remained hope, purpose, and my why—a beacon of light in the darkness guiding me forward into the unknown

A Lifesaving Gesture

As I lay there, my mind reeling from the shock of the accident, the world around me seemed to blur into a haze of noise and confusion. Each passing car felt like a dagger in my heart, their indifference slicing through the air like a chilling wind. I waved frantically, desperately trying to catch someone's attention, but they sped past, their faces nothing but fleeting blurs of indifference.

In my desperation, I turned to whatever resources I had at hand, casting debris onto the road in a desperate attempt to signal for help. My helmet, once my faithful protector, joined the makeshift SOS sign, a silent plea for someone, anyone, to stop and lend a hand. The minutes stretched into eternity, each passing second amplifying the sense of isolation and despair.

And then, like a ray of sunshine breaking through storm clouds, she appeared. An ordinary schoolteacher, her face etched with concern and compassion, stepped out of her car and into my life. In that moment, she wasn't just a stranger; she was a lifeline, a beacon of hope in a sea of uncertainty.

As she knelt beside me and wrapped her arms around me, a sense of relief washed over me like a warm tide. In her embrace, I found solace, a fleeting moment of respite from the chaos and pain that engulfed me. It wasn't about her medical expertise or heroic deeds; it was the simple act of being there, of offering a comforting presence in a moment of desperate need.

For the first time since the accident, I felt a glimmer of hope flicker within me. Despite the pain and uncertainty that lay ahead, I knew that I wasn't alone. In her simple gesture of kindness, she gave me the strength to keep fighting, to cling to the hope that help would come, and that somehow, against all odds, I would make it through.

> *"Embrace uncertainty. Some of the most beautiful chapters in our lives won't have a title until much later."*
> **- Bob Goff, Bestselling Author,
> Honorary Consul to Uganda, Founder of Love Does**

The Brotherhood Arrives

As the minutes stretched on like an eternity, I clung to the edge of despair, each passing second feeling like an eternity. Then, suddenly, the wail of sirens pierced the air, slicing through the suffocating silence like a beacon of hope. My heart leaped with a mixture of relief and gratitude as I watched the fire department's familiar red trucks barrel down the road, their flashing lights cutting through the darkness like a lifeline. In that moment, I felt a surge of reassurance wash over me, knowing that help was finally at hand.

As they rushed to my side, my fellow firefighters brought with them not just medical expertise, but a sense of camaraderie that transcended words. Their presence was a tangible reminder of the bond we shared, forged through countless hours of training and countless calls to serve. Even as they worked to stabilize me, their unwavering support served as a pillar of strength, grounding me in the midst of chaos.

In that moment, I couldn't help but reflect on the countless times I had been on the other side, rushing to the aid of those in need. Now, it was my turn to be the one in need, and the knowledge that my brothers were there for me filled me with a profound sense of gratitude. Despite the pain and uncertainty that gripped me, I felt a sense of reassurance knowing that I was not alone in this battle.

Thoughts raced through my mind in a whirlwind of emotions – gratitude for the swift response of my fellow firefighters, fear for what lay ahead, and a glimmer of hope that I would emerge from this trial stronger than before. With each passing moment, I clung to the support of my brothers, drawing strength from their unwavering presence by my side.

The Unseen Audience

As the ambulance rushed me to the hospital, every jolt and sway amplified the pain pulsing through my body, a relentless reminder of the ordeal I had endured. But amidst the chaos of sirens and flashing lights, I was unaware of the unseen audience that had gathered, their silent prayers and hopes trailing behind me like a comforting blanket.

As we approached the hospital, the scene that greeted me was nothing short of overwhelming. Lined up in a solemn row, my fellow firefighters stood like guardians, their faces etched with concern and determination. Each one was a pillar of support, a testament to the unwavering bond we shared as members of the same family in firefighting.

The chief's words, delivered with quiet authority, echoed through the air, filling me with a sense of belonging and purpose. In that moment, surrounded by my brothers and sisters in uniform, I felt a surge of gratitude and pride, knowing that I was part of something greater than myself.

Thoughts raced through my mind as I took in the sight before me–gratitude for the outpouring of support, a sense of awe at the strength of the human spirit, and a deep-seated determination to overcome whatever challenges lay ahead. Emotions swirled within me like a tempest, mingling fear with hope, uncertainty with resolve.

As I was wheeled into the hospital, I carried with me the collective strength and support of my firefighting family, a beacon of light guiding me through the darkness. This chapter is a testament to the power of resilience, the importance of brotherhood, and the courage we find in the unlikeliest of places.

It's in all of us.

Oxytocin, often referred to as the "love hormone," is a fascinating chemical that plays a crucial role in various aspects of human behavior and physiology. It is released in significant amounts during childbirth, breastfeeding, and parent-child bonding, contributing to the formation of strong emotional connections between individuals. Additionally, oxytocin is involved in promoting trust, empathy, and bonding in social relationships, and its levels tend to increase with physical affection such as kissing, cuddling, and sexual intimacy.

Beyond its role in reproductive processes, oxytocin influences a wide range of psychological and physiological functions. Psychologically, oxytocin is associated with feelings of love, trust, and social bonding. It enhances prosocial behaviors and fosters a sense of connection and closeness with others. Physiologically, oxytocin has been found to have effects on the cardiovascular system, stress regulation, and immune function.

Research has shown that individuals with higher levels of oxytocin tend to exhibit greater generosity, empathy, and willingness to help others. Simple acts of kindness and human generosity can lead to a release of oxytocin, creating a positive feedback loop of prosocial behavior. Moreover, witnessing acts of kindness in others can also elevate oxytocin levels, promoting a ripple effect of compassion and altruism in social networks.

Measuring oxytocin levels in the body typically involves collecting blood or saliva samples and analyzing them for oxytocin concentration. However, it's essential to note that oxytocin levels can fluctuate throughout the day in response to various stimuli and experiences. Factors such as social interactions, stress levels, and physical touch can influence oxytocin release, highlighting the dynamic nature of this hormone.

Incorporating practices that promote oxytocin release into daily life can have significant benefits for overall well-being and inter-personal relationships. Simple activities such as hugging loved ones, engaging in acts of kindness, and spending quality time with friends and family can help boost oxytocin levels. Moreover, practicing mindfulness, engaging in relaxation techniques, and participating in social activities can also contribute to oxytocin release.

Connecting oxytocin to the themes explored in earlier chapters of this book underscores its role in fostering resilience, building strong social connections, and promoting emotional healing. From the support of friends and family during challenging times to the profound bonds formed through shared experiences, oxytocin emerges as a key player in shaping the narrative of human relationships and resilience. By understanding the physiological and psychological mechanisms underlying oxytocin's effects, individuals can harness its power to cultivate compassion, connection, and well-being in their lives.

Emergency Havoc

As I was wheeled through the doors of the emergency room, the chaos engulfed me like a tidal wave, threatening to drown out all sense of calm. The sterile scent of disinfectant mingled with the metallic tang of blood, creating an atmosphere charged with tension and urgency. All around me, figures clad in scrubs darted back and forth, their movements a blur of purpose and determination. Each face I glimpsed seemed to blur into the next, a whirlwind of activity amidst the cacophony of alarms and voices.

The sting of needles piercing my skin was a sharp punctuation to the symphony of chaos, a reminder of the harsh reality of my situation. With each injection, the promise of relief hovered tantalizingly close, yet remained just beyond my grasp. The flood of painkillers that followed was a desperate attempt to silence the relentless roar of agony that reverberated through every fiber of my being. Yet, even as the drugs coursed through my veins, their effects proved fleeting, a temporary respite from the unyielding onslaught of pain.

Amidst the turmoil, the doctor emerged as a beacon of calm amidst the storm, his steady voice cutting through the chaos like a guiding light. With a reassuring hand on my shoulder, he gently proposed the possibility of a medically induced coma—a temporary reprieve from the relentless torment that had become my reality. In that moment, the prospect of escape beckoned like a distant oasis in the desert, offering a glimmer of hope amidst the darkness of my suffering. Desperate for relief, I found myself clinging to his words, willing to embrace any semblance of respite from the unrelenting anguish that threatened to consume me.

In the Realm of Shadows

They ushered me into a realm of unconsciousness that stretched like an eternity, a fleeting respite from the tumultuous world outside. For eight days, I traversed the shadowy expanse of my mind, navigating a labyrinth of dreams and nightmares that blurred the line between reality and illusion. Surgeries came and went like fleeting specters in the night, each one a whispered promise of restoration and renewal.

I remember thinking my brain was shutting down. Like a computer was turning off. I could see the lines across the screen of my mind. I remember thinking, *I am dying*.

As I drifted through the murky depths of unconsciousness, the passage of time became a nebulous concept, its meaning lost in the swirling currents of my subconscious. Yet, amidst the darkness, fragments of awareness flickered like distant stars in the night sky. The sensation of being adrift in an endless sea of oblivion was punctuated only by the rhythmic thrum of machines and the faint echo of voices that seemed to drift in from a distant shore.

And then, like a beacon cutting through the fog, the moment of awakening arrived—a gradual emergence from the depths of oblivion into the harsh light of consciousness. The tube in my throat felt like an anchor tethering me to the realm of the living, its presence a stark reminder of the fragile balance between life and death. And there, amidst the stark sterility of the hospital room, my mother's face shone like a guiding light, a familiar anchor in the sea of uncertainty.

Her gentle words washed over me like a soothing tide, their warmth a lifeline amidst the cold uncertainty of my surroundings.

In her eyes, I found solace and reassurance, a silent testament to the unbreakable bond between mother and child. As the haze of anesthesia began to lift, I became acutely aware of the extent of my injuries—a harsh reality that threatened to engulf me in a tidal wave of despair.

Yet, in the steady gaze of my mother, I found strength and resilience, a silent promise that together, we would weather the storm that lay ahead.

Anatomy of Survival

Bound to the confines of my hospital bed, I found myself ensnared in a web of immobilization, my body a mere shell of its former self. The halo brace encircling my mended leg served as a tangible reminder of the ordeal I had endured—a physical manifestation of the fractures that had threatened to shatter my very existence. Each metal ring pressed against my skin like a silent witness to the fragility of life, their presence a constant reminder of the delicate balance between survival and oblivion.

As my mother's voice washed over me, her words painted a stark portrait of my condition—a portrait etched in the harsh lines of medical jargon and clinical terminology. "Don't move, honey. Your neck is broken in two places, and you broke your back, in three, but you are ok." A litany of injuries that seemed inconceivable in their severity. And yet, as the reality of my plight began to sink in, I found myself grappling with a sense of disbelief—a gnawing uncertainty that gnawed at the edges of my consciousness.

"What are you talking about? How is that possible?"

I had traversed that desolate ditch, fighting tooth and nail for each precious breath, all the while oblivious to the fractures that lurked beneath the surface. The sheer resilience of the human body astounded me, its capacity to endure unimaginable pain and suffering a testament to the indomitable spirit that resides within us all. In the face of such adversity, the will to live emerged as a beacon of hope—a guiding light that pierced through the darkness of despair, illuminating the path to recovery and renewal.

As I lay tethered to my hospital bed, I marveled at the miraculous interplay between mind and body, the intricate dance of healing and transformation that unfolded within the recesses of my being. Though my physical form may have been battered and broken, my spirit remained unbroken—a testament to the unwavering resilience of the human soul. And so, with each passing moment, I resolved to channel that inner strength, to defy the odds and emerge from the shadows of adversity, reborn and renewed.

Days of Dependency

The ensuing days blurred into a haze of uncertainty, each one a testament to the intricate dance between life and death orchestrated by the medical team. In the sterile confines of the hospital room, I lay ensnared in the grip of helplessness, my body a mere vessel at the mercy of those who wielded scalpel and syringe with practiced precision. Dignity, once a stalwart companion, now dwindled into obscurity as the primal instinct for survival eclipsed all else.

Immobile and vulnerable, I found myself teetering on the precipice of despair, grappling with the stark reality of my predicament. Each medical test, each whispered consultation, served as a somber refrain in the dirge of uncertainty that echoed through the halls of the hospital. The silent responses from the limb they fought so valiantly to salvage became a haunting melody, a lament for the uncertain fate that lay in wait.

Amidst the clinical efficiency of the medical procedures, a profound sense of fear took root in the recesses of my mind, its tendrils weaving through the fabric of my consciousness like creeping ivy. Uncertainty became my constant companion, casting a pall over every waking moment as I grappled with the looming specter of rejection—the harrowing realization that my own body was waging war against itself in a desperate bid for survival.

As I lay confined to my hospital bed, engulfed by the sterile whiteness of the room, the shadow of uncertainty loomed large, casting its pall over my fragile existence. Each passing moment brought with it a crescendo of fear and apprehension, a relentless onslaught that threatened to consume me whole. And yet, amidst the darkness, a flicker of resilience emerged—a defiant spark that refused to be extinguished, illuminating the path forward with a glimmer of hope amidst the encroaching gloom.

The Inevitable Verdict

The day the doctor uttered those fateful words, it felt as though the ground had been ripped out from beneath me, leaving me suspended in a void of disbelief and despair. Amputation—a single word that reverberated through the corridors of my mind with a deafening intensity, shattering the fragile illusions of normalcy that I had clung to so desperately. In that solitary moment, the trajectory of my life irrevocably altered, the weight of an uncertain future bearing down upon me with crushing force.

As the doctor's somber pronouncement hung heavy in the air, tears flowed freely, each droplet a poignant reminder of the profound loss that awaited me. It was as though time itself had paused, allowing the gravity of the situation to sink in—a lifetime of memories, dreams, and aspirations condensed into a single, harrowing realization. And yet, amidst the overwhelming flood of emotions, a flicker of resilience ignited within me—a primal instinct to defy the odds, to reclaim agency over my own fate.

In the aftermath of that fateful diagnosis, a newfound sense of determination surged through my veins, eclipsing the despair that threatened to consume me. Yes, I was facing the prospect of losing a part of myself, but I refused to let it define me. With each passing moment, my resolve strengthened, fueled by an unwavering commitment to persevere in the face of adversity. It was a choice—a conscious decision to embrace the challenges ahead with courage and conviction, knowing that within the depths of my spirit, the flame of resilience burned bright.

Fear

Fear is a potent emotion that permeates every aspect of our lives, influencing our thoughts, behaviors, and decisions. It's a primal response ingrained in our biology, designed to protect us from potential threats. Yet, in today's complex world, fear often manifests in ways that hinder rather than safeguard our well-being.

From the moment we enter the world, fear begins to shape our perceptions and responses. As infants, we are born with only two innate fears—the fear of falling and the fear of loud noises. Every other fear we experience throughout life is learned or accepted from external sources. Parents, friends, colleagues, and the media all contribute to the development of our fears, instilling beliefs about what is dangerous or threatening.

The aftermath of significant events, such as 9/11, demonstrates how fear can have far-reaching consequences. In the wake of the tragedy, many individuals became so fearful of flying that they opted for alternative modes of transportation, resulting in an increase in automobile fatalities. This example underscores the power of fear to distort our perceptions of risk and influence our behavior.

At its core, fear is a hormonal response that triggers physiological changes in the body. When confronted with a perceived threat, our heart rate increases, breathing becomes shallow, and our focus narrows. These physical manifestations are part of our body's survival mechanism, designed to prepare us to fight, flee, or freeze in response to danger.

However, while fear may be an instinctual response, our interpretation and response to fear are within our control. When we allow fear to dictate our thoughts and actions, it can become paralyzing, preventing us from taking risks or pursuing our goals. Fear has a way of distorting our perceptions, leading us to see everything through a lens of negativity and limitation.

One of the most insidious aspects of fear is its ability to trigger a cycle of inaction and negativity. When we are consumed by fear, we become stuck in a state of uncertainty, unable to move forward or make progress. This hesitancy can prevent us from seizing opportunities, pursuing our passions, or realizing our full potential.

In contrast, gratitude serves as a powerful antidote to fear. When we cultivate a mindset of gratitude, we shift our focus away from what we lack or fear and toward what we have and appreciate. Gratitude has the remarkable ability to dismantle fear and anger, replacing them with feelings of abundance and contentment. By practicing gratitude, we can disrupt the cycle of fear and open ourselves up to new possibilities and opportunities.

Athletes understand the importance of mindset in overcoming fear and achieving success. Through visualization and mental rehearsal, they train their minds to focus on success rather than failure. Similarly, in business and everyday life, cultivating a resilient mindset is essential for overcoming fear and achieving our goals. By envisioning success, maintaining a positive outlook, and taking decisive action, we can transcend fear and unlock our full potential.

Ultimately, fear is a natural and inevitable part of the human experience. However, by understanding its origins, recognizing its impact, and cultivating a resilient mindset, we can harness its power and use it as a catalyst for growth and transformation. Fear may have once been essential for our survival, but in today's world, it is our ability to overcome fear that allows us to thrive and flourish.

The Choice is Yours

As I grappled with the reality of my situation, I realized that I stood at a crossroads—a pivotal moment where the trajectory of my life hinged on the choices I made. It would have been all too easy to succumb to the depths of despair, to allow the shadows of doubt and fear to envelop me in their suffocating embrace. I could have allowed myself to become a mere shell of my former self, consumed by bitterness and resentment at the hand fate had dealt me.

But deep within the recesses of my being, a spark of determination flickered defiantly—a beacon of hope amidst the darkness. It was a reminder that, even in the face of seemingly insurmountable odds, I still held the power to shape my own destiny. I could choose to wallow in self-pity and anguish, or I could rise above the adversity, embracing it as an opportunity for growth and transformation.

So, I made a choice—a choice to refuse defeat, to embrace the challenges that lay ahead with unwavering resolve. Yes, losing my leg was undoubtedly a devastating blow, but it was also a catalyst for change—a chance to reinvent myself, to discover the depths of my own strength and resilience. Instead of allowing myself to be defined by my circumstances, I chose to redefine them, to carve out a new path filled with purpose and meaning.

In accepting the reality of my situation, I also accepted the challenge—to never lose sight of the fighter within me, to never relinquish the flame of determination that burned fiercely in my soul. It was a conscious decision to confront adversity head-on, to confront it with a spirit of resilience and unwavering determination. And in doing so, I discovered a newfound sense of empowerment—a realization that no matter what life may throw my way, I possess the power to rise above it, to emerge stronger and more resilient than ever before.

Looking Ahead

As I sat there, amidst the whispers of doubt and uncertainty, I felt a surge of determination coursing through my veins. The weight of the moment hung heavy in the air, but I refused to let it crush my spirit. Instead, I turned to my father with a steely resolve, a determination etched into every line of my face.

"Dad, get my tablet and let's find the best prosthetic leg in the world."

In that pivotal moment, as I spoke those words, I realized that I was not just asking for a prosthetic leg—I was demanding a symbol of my resilience, a tangible testament to my unwavering commitment to reclaiming my life. It was a declaration to the world that I refused to be defined by my limitations, that I was determined to defy the odds and rewrite the narrative of my future.

Despite the doubt that lingered in the room, I held fast to the unwavering belief that anything was possible with the right mindset and determination. It was this unwavering conviction that fueled my drive to seek out the best prosthetic leg available, knowing that it would be the key to unlocking a new chapter in my life.

In that moment, I made a silent vow to myself—a vow to not only return to firefighting but to do so with a renewed sense of purpose and passion. I was determined to blaze trails, to shatter stereotypes, and to redefine what it meant to be a firefighter. The road ahead might be daunting, filled with challenges and obstacles, but I was ready to face them head-on, armed with nothing but my sheer determination and unyielding resolve.

Flame of Determination

As I reflect on that momentous decision, I realize the profound importance of having a goal—a beacon of light to guide you through the darkest of times. My goal wasn't just about getting a prosthetic leg; it was about reclaiming my identity, my purpose, and my passion for firefighting. It was about proving to myself and to the world that nothing could extinguish the flame of determination burning within me.

One crucial lesson I learned throughout this journey is the power of persistence. I didn't set an arbitrary timeline for my goal; instead, I committed myself wholeheartedly to the process, understanding that true progress takes time. Every setback, every challenge, only fueled my determination to keep pushing forward, one step at a time.

And let me tell you, that same resilience resides within every one of us. Whether you're facing a physical challenge, a professional setback, or a personal struggle, know that you have the power to overcome it. Set your sights on a goal that ignites your passion and fuels your spirit, and don't let anything deter you from pursuing it relentlessly.

Remember, success is not always about how quickly you achieve your goal; it's about the journey, the resilience, and the unwavering commitment to never give up. So, I urge you, take that first step towards your goal today, and keep moving forward with unwavering determination. Trust me when I say that with persistence, dedication, and a clear vision of what you want to achieve, there's no limit to what you can accomplish.

Discovery and Resolve

In the quiet moments of reflection during my hospital stay, a glimmer of hope emerged—a plan, a path forward toward reclaiming the life I once knew. With unwavering determination, my family and I embarked on a journey to find the perfect prosthetic leg, one that would not only restore mobility but also symbolize resilience and strength.

After thorough research and consultations, we discovered the Ottobock X3, a prosthetic marvel known for its exceptional durability and tailored design for active individuals like myself. It was more than just a prosthetic; it was a beacon of possibility, a symbol of hope for a future filled with new challenges and triumphs.

As I gazed upon the X3, I felt a surge of determination coursing through my veins. This was the leg that would accompany me on my journey back to firefighting, through trials and triumphs alike. It was waterproof, dirt-proof, and seemingly built to withstand the rigors of firefighting—the perfect match for my resilient spirit.

However, amidst the excitement of finding the perfect prosthetic, I was acutely aware of the hurdles that lay ahead. The mere acquisition of the Ottobock X3 was just the first step in a long and arduous process. There were insurance paperwork to navigate, countless hours of rehabilitation and recovery, and the daunting task of learning to walk again. Yet, despite the challenges looming on the horizon, I remained steadfast in my resolve to make the Ottobock X3 an integral part of my life.

Double Amputation

The day following the surgery was a pivotal moment, a crossroads in my life where the trajectory of my journey took an unexpected turn. While the initial operation removed my leg below the knee, the extent of the damage to my knee itself was more severe than anticipated. It became clear that preserving my knee was no longer feasible—it had to be amputated as well. This decision marked a profound shift in my journey, signaling a departure from the path I had envisioned and thrusting me into uncharted territory.

Facing the reality of losing my knee brought with it a wave of uncertainty and apprehension. Without this crucial joint, every aspect of my mobility would be altered, and the prospect of relearning even the most basic movements loomed large. However, in the midst of this uncertainty, I refused to see it as an end. Instead, I embraced it as a new beginning, a chance to redefine my capabilities and rewrite the narrative of my life.

Though the road ahead appeared daunting and filled with challenges, I viewed it as an opportunity for growth and transformation. Each step forward would be a testament to my resilience and determination, a reminder that adversity does not define us but rather shapes us into who we are meant to become. In this pivotal moment, I chose to embrace the unknown with courage and optimism, knowing that within every obstacle lay the seeds of opportunity and renewal.

Rehabilitation: First Steps Reimagined

After undergoing the extensive surgeries, St. Mary's of the Lake Hospital transformed into my battlefield, a place where I embarked on the arduous journey of rediscovering the fundamentals of life. It was here, amidst the sterile halls and bustling corridors, that I confronted the daunting task of rebuilding my physical strength and mobility from the ground up. Each day presented a new set of challenges, from simply sitting up without feeling dizzy to gradually gaining the confidence to stand unaided.

The process was undeniably humbling, as I found myself back at square one, grappling with tasks that once seemed effortless. Yet, amid the frustration and setbacks, there was a glimmer of familiarity—a recognition that I had faced similar obstacles before and emerged stronger each time. This resilience, rooted deep within me, became the driving force propelling me forward in the face of adversity.

Guided by the compassionate therapists at St. Mary's, I embarked on a journey of self-discovery and empowerment. Their expertise provided me with invaluable guidance and support, but it was ultimately my own unwavering determination that propelled me toward progress. Together, we navigated the challenges of rehabilitation, each session serving as a stepping stone toward reclaiming my independence and autonomy.

Pushing Boundaries

Day by day, I embarked on a relentless pursuit to challenge my own boundaries, pushing against the constraints of my physical limitations with unwavering determination. The prosthetic leg, once a symbol of loss and adversity, gradually transformed into an emblem of resilience and strength, serving as a tangible manifestation of my indomitable willpower. It was no longer merely a functional aid but rather an extension of my inner resolve, propelling me forward on my journey of recovery and self-discovery.

My pursuit was not driven solely by a desire to return to a sense of normalcy; it was fueled by an insatiable thirst to surpass even the loftiest of expectations. In the face of skepticism and doubt, I refused to conform to perceived limitations, setting my sights on lofty goals that defied conventional wisdom. When others suggested a modest thirty, I defiantly pushed myself to achieve three hundred, demonstrating a steadfast commitment to exceed not only others' expectations but also my own.

This relentless drive propelled me back into the familiar surroundings of the gym, where I embraced the challenges of rigorous training with a renewed sense of purpose. Each session became an opportunity to test the boundaries of my physical capabilities, to defy the odds stacked against me, and to inch closer toward reclaiming my former strength and vitality. Despite the initial setbacks and hurdles, I remained undeterred in my pursuit of progress, determined to prove that resilience knows no bounds.

The Chief's Challenge

The anticipation of my imminent return to active duty reverberated through the corridors of the fire station, igniting a palpable buzz of excitement and curiosity. As rumors of my readiness reached the ears of the chief, his inquiry hung in the air like a weighty challenge, daring me to prove my mettle. With unwavering confidence born from months of arduous rehabilitation and relentless determination, I met his question with a resounding affirmation—a silent vow to myself and to all who stood witness to my journey.

The chief's question wasn't merely an inquiry; it was a pivotal moment of validation—an acknowledgment of my readiness to reclaim my rightful place among my fellow firefighters. It was a chance not only to demonstrate my physical capability but also to reaffirm my commitment to the unwavering brotherhood that bound us together. In that moment, I recognized that this opportunity was more than just a return to duty; it was a testament to the resilience of the human spirit and the power of collective solidarity.

As I prepared to re-enter the fray, I found solace in the unwavering support of my colleagues—the brothers and sisters who had stood by my side throughout the darkest days of my journey. Together, we embarked on a shared mission, fueled by a common purpose and a shared determination to uphold the values that defined us as firefighters. In their camaraderie, I found strength; in their encouragement, I found resolve; and in their unwavering belief in my abilities, I found the courage to confront the challenges that lay ahead.

United by the unbreakable bond of our shared experiences and our shared commitment to the noble calling of firefighting, we stood shoulder to shoulder, ready to face whatever trials awaited us. In that moment, the fire that burned within us blazed brighter than ever before, casting aside any doubts or uncertainties that lingered in the recesses of our minds. For we knew that together, as a unified force, we were capable of overcoming any obstacle, surmounting any challenge, and emerging victorious in the pursuit of our collective mission.

A Milestone Achieved

And then, like a beacon of light piercing through the darkest of nights, a milestone that once seemed as distant as the stars was suddenly within my grasp. The impending test day loomed over me like a looming storm cloud, casting shadows of doubt and uncertainty across my path. What if I didn't pass? The question echoed relentlessly in the chambers of my mind, its persistent whispers threatening to undermine the unwavering resolve that had carried me thus far.

Yet, despite the gnawing apprehension that coiled in the pit of my stomach, I couldn't help but feel a flicker of excitement—a palpable anticipation that tingled in the air like static electricity before a thunderstorm. Never before had I felt such a potent mix of nerves and readiness, a cocktail of emotions that surged through my veins with an intensity that eclipsed even the fiercest competition on the sports field.

For this test, this challenge, was more than just a mere checkpoint on my journey—it was a defining moment, a culmination of years of tireless effort, relentless perseverance, and unyielding determination. It was a testament to my identity, my purpose, my very essence as a firefighter—a calling that had become synonymous with my being, inseparable from the core of my existence.

As the hours ticked by and the fateful moment drew near, I found myself standing on the precipice of destiny, my heart pounding like a drumbeat in my chest. But amidst the whirlwind of emotions that threatened to engulf me, there was a quiet confidence—a steadfast belief that I had prepared, that I had trained, that I was ready.

"Mike, ready?.......Go!"

I shot up the first flight of stairs like I was invincible. No thought of my physical situation. I pulled the rope like I was reeling in a fishing line. I grabbed the SmartDummy Extrication Manikin like a stuff animal and dragged it across the line. I was exhausted, but I only had one goal.

As the final bell tolled and the dust settled, the truth revealed itself. Did I pass? Did I triumph over doubt, over fear, over every obstacle that had dared to stand in my way? At that moment, as the weight of my achievement settled upon my shoulders like a crown of victory, I dropped to my knees in exhaustion while a flood of emotion got the best of me. I cried, and laughed — I knew with unwavering certainty that I had become Canada's first full-time above-knee amputated firefighter.

But this victory was not mine alone—it belonged to every person who has ever faced the impossible and dared to push forward. It was a testament to the indomitable spirit of the human soul, a reminder that true strength is not measured by the absence of adversity, but by the courage to confront it head-on and emerge victorious on the other side. And so, as I stood there, bathed in the warm glow of accomplishment, I knew that this was not just the end of one chapter, but the beginning of an extraordinary journey—a journey fueled by hope, fueled by resilience, fueled by the unwavering belief that anything is possible if we dare to dream.

Summary

Chapter 4 stands as a testament to the resilience of the human spirit, a narrative woven with the threads of tragedy and triumph that altered the trajectory of my life forever. It begins with the roar of a motorcycle engine, the wind in my hair, and the promise of adventure on the horizon. Yet, in the blink of an eye, that promising journey takes a dark turn when a collision with a deer shatters the tranquility of the ride, propelling me into a harrowing crash that left me with severe injuries, including the loss of my leg—a sudden and cruel twist of fate that would test my resolve in ways I could never have imagined.

In the aftermath of the accident, amidst the wreckage of broken bones and shattered dreams, emerges a glimmer of hope in the form of the Ottobock X3 prosthetic leg—a beacon of possibility in a sea of uncertainty. This state-of-the-art limb symbolizes more than just a physical replacement; it embodies the promise of reclaiming my identity as a firefighter, of regaining the sense of purpose that had defined me for so long. Despite the daunting prospect of complex surgeries and the stark reality of facing life with an above-knee amputation, my determination remains unyielding, a steadfast flame that refuses to be extinguished by the darkness of despair.

Rehabilitation becomes my battleground, where every step is a victory and every setback a challenge to overcome. It is a journey fraught with physical pain and mental anguish, where the simple act of sitting up or standing become monumental achievements in themselves. But within the confines of the hospital room, amidst the whirring of machines and the sterile scent of antiseptic, I discover a newfound resilience—an inner strength that propels me forward even when the odds seem insurmountable.

With each passing day, I push the boundaries of what I believed was possible, defying the limitations imposed by my injuries and refusing to be defined by my circumstances. Guided by the unwavering support of physiotherapists and fueled by a personal drive that burned brighter than any flame, I embark on a journey of self-discovery and transformation—a journey that will redefine the very essence of recovery.

The culmination of this arduous odyssey is nothing short of miraculous—a triumphant return to the fire department, a testament to the power of perseverance and the resilience of the human spirit. Though initially relegated to light duties, my ambition burned undiminished, fueled by a determination to reclaim my rightful place among my comrades. And in a moment that defied all expectations, a year after the accident, I shattered barriers and made history as Canada's first full-time above-knee amputated firefighter—a living testament to the unyielding power of courage, perseverance, and an unwavering will to overcome.

Chapter 4

From Solace to Romance

"Sometimes it takes a wrong turn to get you to the right place."
~ **Mandy Hale**, bestselling author known for her inspirational writings on personal empowerment.

4

Hospital Days and Nights

I bid farewell to the sterile confines of the ICU, trading the rhythmic beeps of monitors for the hushed whispers of the longer, quieter halls of St. Mary's of the Lake Hospital. It was a transition into a new world, one where the scent of antiseptic mingled with the warmth of familiarity, and the hospital staff became like family. As the days stretched into weeks, I became an inhabitant of this second home, navigating its corridors with the ease of a seasoned traveler.

Physiotherapy sessions punctuated my days, each one a step closer to reclaiming the mobility I had lost. From the gentle guidance of therapists to the camaraderie of fellow patients, every interaction became a source of strength and resilience. And in the stillness of the night, when sleep eluded me and the ceiling tiles became my only companions, I discovered solace in the simplicity of movement.

Amidst the quiet hum of machinery and the distant echoes of others' pain, I found moments of levity that broke through the monotony of hospital life. Simple exercises from my hospital bed became miniature triumphs, each movement a victory in its own right. Whether it was the satisfaction of reaching a new milestone or the shared laughter with fellow patients, these small moments of joy illuminated the darkest corners of my hospital room.

But amidst the routine of physiotherapy and the monotony of hospital life, there were also moments of unexpected humor that brought levity to the most challenging of circumstances. From the antics of fellow patients to the lighthearted banter with nurses, laughter became a balm for the soul—a reminder that even in the face of adversity, there is room for joy.

As I navigated the halls of St. Mary's of the Lake Hospital, I discovered that resilience often comes not from the grand gestures, but from the small, everyday triumphs. And in embracing the humor and humanity of hospital life, I found a newfound sense of strength and resilience that would carry me through the challenges that lay ahead.

Unexpected Crossroads of Fate

Amidst the backdrop of healing and recovery, there were moments of unexpected levity that injected a sense of whimsy into the otherwise sterile corridors of the hospital. As I navigated the halls in my wheelchair, I found myself embracing the role of a speedster, careening around corners with the clatter of my IV pole keeping rhythm. It was a scene straight out of a slapstick comedy, and I couldn't help but find humor in the absurdity of it all. Remember the movie Joe Dirt? Now, amputate his leg, throw him in a wheelchair, and imagine him in a beautiful two-tone ocean blue hospital gown….sexy!

Despite the gravity of my situation, I found myself craving a reprieve from the monotony of hospital life—a distraction from the clinical routines and the relentless beeping of machines. And so, in a state that resembled less a firefighter and more a character out of a comedy, I embarked on an unlikely quest for romance.

One might question the timing of such pursuits, but amidst the stark surroundings of the hospital, I couldn't ignore the longing for connection, for a spark of warmth amidst the clinical coldness. And it was in the midst of this search that I stumbled upon her—a nurse whose presence was like a beacon of light in the dimly lit corridors.

From the moment our eyes met, I knew there was something different about her. It wasn't just her arresting beauty or the gentle kindness in her eyes; it was something deeper, something that resonated with the very core of my being. In that instant, amidst the chaos of hospital life, I felt a connection unlike any I had experienced before—a connection that transcended the confines of illness and injury.

As I watched her move gracefully through the ward, tending to patients with a warmth and compassion that was palpable, I couldn't help but be drawn to her. It was as if fate had intervened, bringing us together in the most unlikely of circumstances—a collision of two souls on parallel paths, converging in the most unexpected of ways.

And so, amidst the whirlwind of hospital life, a love story began to unfold—a story that would defy the odds and stand as a testament to the power of love in the face of adversity. For in that moment, as I gazed into her eyes, I knew that I had found something worth fighting for—a love that would light the way through the darkest of nights.

From Hospital to Happily Ever After

We exchanged pleasantries, our names becoming the first brushstrokes on the canvas of our budding connection. As I wheeled back to my room, the thought of reaching out on Facebook lingered in my mind—a digital lifeline cast into the vast expanse of uncertainty, in the hopes that she would see beyond the confines of the hospital and into the essence of who I truly was.

With trembling fingers, I sent the friend request, half-hoping and half-dreading the outcome. It was a small gesture, a tentative step into the unknown, but little did I know that it would set the stage for a journey that would change the course of my life.

Days turned into weeks, and weeks into months, each passing moment a testament to the resilience of the human spirit and the power of hope. Through the arduous process of rehabilitation, I rediscovered the strength within myself, inching closer to the life I once knew and the dreams I dared to envision.

With each tentative step on my new prosthetic leg, I felt the weight of my past struggles begin to lift, replaced by a sense of newfound freedom and possibility. And as I regained my footing in the world, a simple question hung in the air, waiting to be answered: Would you like to go on a date?

It was a question that held the promise of a future filled with hope and possibility, a chance to rewrite the narrative of my life and embrace the love that had found its way into my heart. And so, with bated breath and a heart full of anticipation, I awaited her response.

The days passed in a blur of excitement and uncertainty, until finally, the answer came—a resounding yes that echoed through the corridors of my soul, filling me with a sense of joy and possibility.

Our first date was simple yet profound—a shared cup of coffee, a leisurely walk through the hospital grounds, and an overeager confession of dreams and aspirations. It was a moment frozen in time, a snapshot of two souls connecting in the most unexpected of places.

But fate, it seems, had other plans. In the days that followed, silence descended like a shroud, leaving me to wonder if our connection had been nothing more than a fleeting moment in time. Yet, even as doubt gnawed at the edges of my consciousness, a glimmer of hope remained—a belief that our story was far from over.

And then, like a twist of fate, our paths crossed once more, setting the stage for a love story that would defy the odds and stand as a testament to the power of perseverance and faith.

In October 2018, we embarked on a new chapter of our journey as husband and wife, our hearts intertwined in a bond that transcended time and space. Together, we navigated the highs and lows of life, embracing the joy of parenthood with the arrival of our little boy, Lincoln, and the vibrant energy of my stepdaughter, Keiana, who is a highly functioning child with Down syndrome.

Our house in Kingston became more than just a place to call home; it became a symbol of our resilience and our unwavering belief in the possibility of second chances. Piece by piece, chance by chance, we rebuilt our lives into something extraordinary—a testament to the transformative power of love and the enduring strength of the human spirit.

And as we stand on the threshold of our future, hand in hand, I am reminded that sometimes, the greatest moments of our lives come from the most unexpected crossroads of fate—leading us not just to happiness, but to a love that knows no bounds.

Chapter 5

Never Stop Climbing

"If you want to go fast, go along. If you want to go far, go together."
~ African Proverb

5

Connecting the Dots

Throughout my book, I have explored themes of resilience, adversity, and personal growth, all of which are intricately linked to the concepts of significance and connection. From my experiences as a firefighter to my journey of recovery, these themes have underscored the importance of human connection in overcoming challenges and finding meaning in life.

In each chapter, I have shared personal anecdotes, insights, and reflections that highlight the transformative power of connection. Whether recounting moments of camaraderie with my fellow firefighters or reflecting on the impact of virtual connections during the pandemic, I have emphasized the role of human connection in shaping our experiences and shaping our identities.

As you have journeyed through the pages of my book, I hope you will gain a deeper understanding of the fundamental human needs for significance and connection. By recognizing the importance of these needs in our own lives and in the lives of others, we can cultivate greater empathy, compassion, and resilience. Ultimately, it is through our connections with others that we find purpose, meaning, and fulfillment in life.

The Need for Significance

The innate desire to feel special or unique is deeply ingrained in the human psyche. From the moment we enter the world, we seek validation and recognition from those around us, fueling our sense of self-worth and identity. Even individuals who appear outwardly tough or resilient harbor a need for significance, albeit expressed in different ways.

As social beings, our need for significance extends beyond mere acknowledgment; it encompasses a profound longing to feel valued and appreciated by others. Whether in the workplace or within personal relationships, recognition serves as a powerful motivator, driving us to excel and achieve our goals. When our efforts are acknowledged and celebrated, we experience a surge of positive emotions, including serotonin, oxytocin, and dopamine, which further reinforce our sense of significance.

In the workplace, recognition takes various forms, from verbal praise to tangible rewards such as promotions or bonuses. These gestures not only validate our contributions but also foster a sense of belonging and camaraderie within the team. Conversely, a lack of recognition can lead to feelings of disillusionment and disengagement, undermining morale and productivity.

Leaders who understand the importance of significance in motivating their employees are better equipped to cultivate a positive work environment. By acknowledging and celebrating individual achievements, they foster a culture of appreciation and empowerment, resulting in higher levels of job satisfaction and performance.

Similarly, in personal relationships, expressions of gratitude and acknowledgment play a vital role in strengthening bonds and fostering intimacy. When we feel seen, heard, and valued by our loved ones, we experience a deep sense of connection and belonging. Conversely, neglecting to express appreciation can erode trust and intimacy, leading to feelings of resentment and dissatisfaction.

Understanding and fulfilling each other's need for significance is essential for building healthy and fulfilling relationships. By demonstrating appreciation and recognition, we affirm our loved ones' value and reinforce the bonds of trust and affection that bind us together.

The Need for Connection

The need for connection lies at the heart of the human experience, driving us to seek love, belonging, and companionship. As social creatures, we are hardwired to form connections with others, as these relationships provide us with emotional support, validation, and a sense of belonging.

In today's digital age, social media platforms have become lifelines for maintaining connections, particularly during times of isolation and upheaval. The COVID-19 pandemic underscored the importance of virtual connections in bridging physical distances and sustaining social bonds. However, while digital communication offers a semblance of connection, nothing can replace the intimacy and warmth of face-to-face interaction.

The concept of connection extends beyond mere social interactions; it encompasses a deep sense of belonging and community. Whether within a family, team, or organization, strong connections foster a sense of unity and shared purpose, enabling individuals to weather challenges and achieve collective goals.

For me, as a firefighter, the bonds forged with my colleagues were integral to my resilience and recovery following traumatic accidents. The sense of camaraderie and mutual support within the firefighting community provided me with strength and solace during some of the darkest moments of my life. In turn, my identity as a firefighter imbued me with a profound sense of purpose and significance, driving me to overcome adversity and continue serving others.

The connections we form with others not only shape our sense of identity but also influence our behaviors and decisions. As I navigated through the aftermath of my accidents, I felt a deep sense of responsibility towards my colleagues, friends, and loved ones, knowing that my actions and choices would impact their lives as well.

In my journey of recovery and self-discovery, I came to appreciate the interconnectedness of human experience and the profound impact of genuine connections. Whether in times of crisis or moments of joy, our connections with others sustain us, uplift us, and remind us of the inherent value of human connection.

Make Yourself Laugh

Making yourself laugh, even without a specific reason, can have profound effects on your mood and well-being. The simple act of laughing triggers the release of feel-good brain chemicals, such as endorphins, which elevate your mood and reduce stress levels.

During my time in the hospital, there were days when the weight of my injuries and the uncertainty of the future threatened to overwhelm me. In those moments, I turned to laughter as a form of self-care. Whether I found humor in silly jokes, funny YouTube videos, or memories of past adventures, the act of laughing provided a much-needed respite from the challenges I faced.

I vividly recall moments spent laughing with Jarrett, one of my closest friends, a confidant, and co-author of this book, during those difficult days. His infectious laughter and witty humor never failed to lift my spirits and remind me that joy could still be found amidst adversity. Even now, whenever I need a pick-me-up, I know I can count on Jarrett to bring a smile to my face and lighten the heaviest of burdens.

Short-Term Benefits

The short-term benefits of laughter extend beyond mere amusement; they encompass a range of physiological and psychological effects that promote overall well-being. Laughter stimulates vital organs, enhances oxygen intake, and releases endorphins, all of which contribute to a sense of happiness and relaxation.

During my recovery, I witnessed firsthand how laughter could transform the atmosphere within the hospital walls. Whether it was sharing funny stories with fellow patients or joking with nurses and doctors, moments of laughter brought a sense of warmth and camaraderie to an otherwise sterile environment. These interactions not only provided temporary relief from pain and discomfort but also fostered connections that buoyed my spirits and fueled my determination to heal.

Laughing Will Soothe Tension

Laughter has a remarkable ability to soothe tension and alleviate stress, both physically and emotionally. By increasing oxygen-rich air to the body and stimulating circulation, laughter promotes muscle relaxation and reduces the physical symptoms of stress.

During my recovery, there were countless moments when laughter served as a lifeline, helping me navigate through moments of intense pain and frustration. Whether it was a witty remark from a nurse or a lighthearted exchange with a fellow patient, laughter offered a welcome reprieve from the challenges I faced. It reminded me that even in the darkest of times, there was still light and laughter to be found.

Long-Term Effects

The long-term effects of laughter extend far beyond momentary relief; they encompass profound benefits for both physical and mental health. Laughter has been shown to boost the immune system, alleviate pain, and improve overall well-being.

As I reflect on my journey of recovery, I am struck by the profound impact that laughter has had on my resilience and outlook on life. Despite facing numerous setbacks and obstacles, laughter has remained a constant source of strength and optimism. Whether it's sharing a joke with a friend or finding humor in everyday moments, laughter has been instrumental in helping me cope with difficult situations and maintain a positive mindset.

Increase Personal Satisfaction

In addition to its physical and emotional benefits, laughter plays a crucial role in fostering social connections and enhancing personal satisfaction. Laughter brings people together, forging bonds of friendship and camaraderie that transcend adversity.

Throughout my recovery, I have been blessed with the unwavering support of friends, family, and colleagues who have stood by my side through the darkest of times. Their laughter and companionship have been a source of comfort and joy, reminding me that I am never alone in my journey.

Laughter is not just a fleeting moment of amusement; it is a powerful tool for healing, resilience, and connection. By embracing laughter and surrounding ourselves with people who make us smile, we can navigate life's challenges with grace, optimism, and joy.

Unwavering Support

In reflecting on the past two decades of my life, I am reminded of a poignant saying about friendship that resonates deeply with me: 'A good friend: Calls you in jail. A great friend: Bails you out of jail. YOUR BEST FRIEND: Sits next to you while saying "Holy shit, wasn't that fun!?"' This saying encapsulates the essence of the unwavering support and love I have received from those closest to me throughout my journey.

First and foremost, my parents, my pillars of strength and unwavering support, have been my guiding lights through the darkest of times. Their love knows no bounds, and their presence in my life has been a constant source of comfort and inspiration.

But it wasn't just my parents who stood by me. Friends, teammates, family members, colleagues, captains, chiefs, doctors, nurses, and even people from the gym—all rallied around me with unwavering support and love. Their visits, calls, and messages brought a sense of warmth and reassurance during my darkest days.

However, amidst the sea of visitors, there were two notable absences—Jarrett and Jon. Despite their physical absence during my time in the hospital, their presence in my life has been invaluable. Jarrett, my co-author and confidant, has always had a knack for finding the silver lining in any situation, reminding me to find reasons to smile even in the face of adversity. And Jon, who may have only made a brief appearance at the hospital, has demonstrated his unwavering loyalty and support in countless other ways, proving that true friendship transcends physical presence.

One particular incident stands out vividly in my memory—a night in Gananoque, Ontario, where I found myself in a situation that was far from safe. Despite my fears and uncertainty, I reached out to Jonathan, knowing that he would come to my aid without hesitation. True to form, he dropped everything and drove three hours in the middle of the night to be by my side, simply because he knew I needed him. It's moments like these that reaffirm the depth of our friendship and the power of unconditional support.

In hindsight, I realize that true friendship, love, and support come in myriad forms. Whether it's a comforting presence in a hospital room, a reassuring phone call in the dead of night, or a spontaneous act of kindness in a moment of need, the bonds we share with those closest to us have the power to uplift and inspire us in ways we never thought possible.

As I look back on the unwavering support I received from my loved ones, I am filled with gratitude and awe. Their love and encouragement have propelled me forward, inspiring me to triumph over adversity and embrace the journey ahead with renewed strength and resilience. Truly, I am blessed to have such incredible friends and family in my corner, and their unwavering presence in my life is a testament to the enduring power of love and friendship.

Hunter S. Thompson was an American journalist and author. He rose to prominence with the publication of Hell's Angels, a book for which he spent a year living with the Hells Angels motorcycle club to write a first-hand account of their lives and experiences.

As I reflect on the journey I've shared, I'm reminded of the words of Hunter S. Thompson, whose fearless approach to life resonates deeply with my own experiences. At 43, I stand at the threshold of a new chapter, filled with anticipation and possibility. Thompson's sentiment encapsulates the essence of my life thus far – a wild ride filled with twists and turns, highs and lows, but above all, a journey marked by resilience, growth, and an unwavering zest for life. As I look ahead, I am filled with gratitude for the challenges overcome, the lessons learned, and the connections forged along the way. So here's to embracing the chaos, seizing every moment, and living life with unbridled passion and purpose. Because in the end, it's not about arriving safely, but rather about embracing the exhilarating ride and shouting to the world, "Wow! What a ride!'"

"Life should not be a journey to the grave with the intention of arriving safely in a pretty and well preserved body, but rather to skid in broadside in a cloud of smoke, thoroughly used up, totally worn out, and loudly proclaiming "Wow! What a Ride!"